Novel PET Radiotracers with Potential Clinical Applications

Editors

NEIL VASDEV
ABASS ALAVI

PET CLINICS

www.pet.theclinics.com

Consulting Editor
ABASS ALAVI

July 2017 • Volume 12 • Number 3

ELSEVIER

1600 John F. Kennedy Boulevard • Suite 1800 • Philadelphia, Pennsylvania, 19103-2899

http://www.pet.theclinics.com

PET CLINICS Volume 12, Number 3
July 2017 ISSN 1556-8598, ISBN-13: 978-0-323-53144-3

Editor: John Vassallo (j.vassallo@elsevier.com)
Developmental Editor: Meredith Madeira

PET Clinics (ISSN 1556-8598) is published quarterly by Elsevier Inc., 360 Park Avenue South, New York, NY 10010-1710. Months of issue are January, April, July, and October. Periodicals postage paid at New York, NY, and additional mailing offices. Subscription prices per year are $232.00 (US individuals), $381.00 (US institutions), $100.00 (US students), $263.00 (Canadian individuals), $428.00 (Canadian institutions), $140.00 (Canadian students), $268.00 (foreign individuals), $428.00 (foreign institutions), and $140.00 (foreign students). To receive student and resident rate, orders must be accompanied by name of affiliated institution, date of term, and the signature of program/residency coordinator on institution letterhead. Orders will be billed at individual rate until proof of status is received. Foreign air speed delivery is included in all Clinics subscription prices. All prices are subject to change without notice. POSTMASTER: Send address changes to PET Clinics, Elsevier Health Sciences Division, Subscription Customer Service, 3251 Riverport Lane, Maryland Heights, MO 63043. **Customer Service: 1-800-654-2452 (U.S. and Canada); 314-447-8871 (outside U.S. and Canada). Fax: 314-447-8029. E-mail: journalscustomerservice-usa@elsevier.com (for print support); journalsonlinesupport-usa@elsevier.com (for online support).**

Reprints. For copies of 100 or more of articles in this publication, please contact the Commercial Reprints Department, Elsevier Inc., 360 Park Avenue South, New York, NY 10010-1710. Tel.: 212-633-3874; Fax: 212-633-3820; E-mail: reprints@elsevier.com.

PET Clinics is covered in MEDLINE/PubMed (Index Medicus).

Contributors

CONSULTING EDITOR

**ABASS ALAVI, MD, MD (Hon), PhD (Hon),
DSc (Hon)**
Professor of Radiology and Neurology, Division
of Nuclear Medicine, Department of Radiology,
Hospital of the University of Pennsylvania,
University of Pennsylvania Perelman School of
Medicine, Philadelphia, Pennsylvania

EDITORS

NEIL VASDEV, PhD
Director of Radiochemistry, Massachusetts
General Hospital, Associate Professor of
Radiology, Division of Nuclear Medicine and
Molecular Imaging, Harvard Medical School,
Boston, Massachusetts

**ABASS ALAVI, MD, MD (Hon), PhD (Hon),
DSc (Hon)**
Professor of Radiology and Neurology, Division
of Nuclear Medicine, Department of Radiology,
Hospital of the University of Pennsylvania,
University of Pennsylvania Perelman School of
Medicine, Philadelphia, Pennsylvania

AUTHORS

WEIQI BAO, MD, PhD
Attending Physician, PET Center,
Huanshan Hospital, Fudan University,
Shanghai, China

RICHARD P. BAUM, Prof, MD, PhD
Theranostics Center for Molecular
Radiotherapy and Molecular Imaging, Bad
Berka, Germany

ZHENGXIN CAI, PhD
Associate Research Scientist, Department of
Radiology and Biomedical Imaging, PET
Center, Yale University School of Medicine,
New Haven, Connecticut

RICHARD E. CARSON, PhD
Professor, Department of Radiology and
Biomedical Imaging, PET Center, Yale
University School of Medicine, New Haven,
Connecticut

BRADFORD C. DICKERSON, MD
Associate Professor, Frontotemporal
Disorders Unit, Department of Neurology,
Massachusetts General Hospital, Harvard
University, Boston, Massachusetts

GEORGES EL FAKHRI, PhD
Director, Gordon Center for Medical Imaging,
Department of Radiology, Massachusetts
General Hospital, Professor, Department of
Radiology, Harvard Medical School, Boston,
Massachusetts

SJOERD FINNEMA, PhD
Associate Research Scientist, Department of
Radiology and Biomedical Imaging, PET
Center, Yale University School of Medicine,
New Haven, Connecticut

MICHAEL A. GORIN, MD
Department of Urology, The James Buchanan
Brady Urological Institute, Johns Hopkins
University School of Medicine, Baltimore,
Maryland

KELLY E. HENRY, PhD
Department of Radiology, Memorial Sloan
Kettering Cancer Center, New York, New York

YIYUN HENRY HUANG, PhD
Professor, Department of Radiology and
Biomedical Imaging, PET Center, Yale
University School of Medicine, New Haven,
Connecticut

HONGMEI JIA, PhD
Associate Professor, Key Laboratory of
Radiopharmaceuticals, Ministry of Education,
College of Chemistry, Beijing Normal
University, Beijing, China

ANDREAS KJAER, MD, PhD, DMSc
Professor, Department of Clinical Physiology,
Nuclear Medicine & PET, Cluster for Molecular
Imaging Rigshospitalet and University of
Copenhagen, Copenhagen, Denmark

HARSHAD KULKARNI, MD
Theranostics Center for Molecular
Radiotherapy and Molecular Imaging,
Bad Berka, Germany

JASON S. LEWIS, PhD
Department of Radiology, Memorial Sloan
Kettering Cancer Center; Program in Molecular
Pharmacology and Chemistry, Memorial Sloan
Kettering Cancer Center, New York, New York

THEODOSIA MAINA, PhD
Molecular Radiopharmacy, INRASTES, NCSR
"Demokritos", Athens, Greece

JEFFREY MEYER, MD, PhD, FRCP(C)
Canada Research Chair in Neurochemistry of
Depression, Head, Neurochemical Imaging
Program in Mood Disorders, Research Imaging
Centre, Campbell Family Mental Health
Research Institute, Centre for Addiction and
Mental Health, Professor, Department of
Psychiatry, University of Toronto, Toronto,
Ontario, Canada

BERTHOLD A. NOCK, PhD
Molecular Radiopharmacy, INRASTES, NCSR
"Demokritos", Athens, Greece

MORTEN PERSSON, MSc, PhD
CEO, Curasight, Copenhagen, Denmark

MARTIN G. POMPER, MD, PhD
The Russell H. Morgan Department of
Radiology and Radiological Science, Johns
Hopkins University School of Medicine,
Baltimore, Maryland

YOTHIN RAKVONGTHAI, PhD
Division of Nuclear Medicine, Department of
Radiology, Faculty of Medicine, Chulalongkorn
University, Bangkok, Thailand

STEVEN P. ROWE, MD, PhD
The Russell H. Morgan Department of
Radiology and Radiological Science, Johns
Hopkins University School of Medicine,
Baltimore, Maryland

AVIRAL SINGH, MD
Theranostics Center for Molecular
Radiotherapy and Molecular Imaging, Bad
Berka, Germany

DORTHE SKOVGAARD, MD, PhD
Department of Clinical Physiology, Nuclear
Medicine & PET, Cluster for Molecular Imaging
Rigshospitalet and University of Copenhagen,
Copenhagen, Denmark

GARY A. ULANER, MD, PhD
Department of Radiology, Memorial Sloan
Kettering Cancer Center, Weill Cornell Medical
College, New York, New York

CHENJIE XIA, MD
Assistant Professor, Department of Neurology,
Jewish General Hospital, McGill University,
Montreal, Québec, Canada

Contents

Increased human epidermal growth factor receptor 2 (HER2) expression is a hallmark of aggressive breast cancer. Imaging modalities have the potential to diagnose HER2-positive breast cancer and detect distant metastases. The heterogeneity of HER2 expression between primary and metastatic disease sites limits the value of tumor biopsies. Molecular imaging is a noninvasive tool to assess HER2-positive primary lesions and metastases. Radiolabeled antibodies, antibody fragments, and affibody molecules devise a reliable and quantitative method for detecting HER2-positive cancer using PET. HER2-targeted PET imaging is a valuable clinical tool with respect to both the care and maintenance of patients with breast cancer.

Prostate-specific membrane antigen (PSMA) has been explored as a target for molecular imaging of prostate cancer and other malignancies that express PSMA in their tumor-associated neovasculature. Although several PSMA-targeted radiotracers labeled with a variety of radionuclides have been reported, positron-emitting radiotracers labeled with ^{18}F are of particular interest. One such compound, the small molecule PSMA inhibitor [^{18}F]DCFPyL, has demonstrated initial success. This article reviews the literature on this radiotracer, including radiosynthetic approaches to the molecule, data that are available from preclinical experiments, and evidence to date of the clinical utility of this agent in prostate cancer and clear cell renal cell carcinoma.

Gastrin-releasing peptide receptors (GRPRs) represent attractive targets for cancer diagnosis and therapy owing to their overexpression in widespread human tumors. Bombesin (BBN) analogues coupled to suitable chelators for stable radiometal binding have been proposed for diagnostic imaging and radionuclide therapy (theranostics) of GRPR-positive tumors. Recently, interest has shifted from BBN-like receptor agonists to GRPR-radioantagonists, because radioantagonists do not induce adverse effects after injection to patients and display superior pharmacokinetic in vivo profiles. Thus, they seem more advantageous for clinical use compared to agonists. Newer developments highlighting the theranostic potential of GRPR-radioantagonists in cancer patient management are presented herein.

Urokinase plasminogen activator receptor (uPAR) is a key component in proteolysis and extracellular matrix degradation during cancer invasion and metastasis. uPAR overexpression is an important biomarker for aggressiveness in several solid tumors and provides independent clinical information. A recent major breakthrough was obtained with human translation of uPAR PET using ^{68}Ga-NOTA-AE105. Clinical results are encouraging and several large-scale clinical trials are now ongoing. This review focuses on uPAR PET with ^{68}Ga-NOTA-AE105 as a new broadly applicable diagnostic and prognostic imaging biomarker in cancer.

Motion degrades image quality and quantitation of PET images, and is an obstacle to quantitative PET imaging. Simultaneous PET-MR offers a tool that can be used for correcting the motion in PET images by using anatomic information from MR imaging acquired concurrently. Motion correction can be performed by transforming a set of reconstructed PET images into the same frame or by incorporating the transformation into the system model and reconstructing the motion-corrected image. Several phantom and patient studies have validated that MR-based motion correction strategies have great promise for quantitative PET imaging in simultaneous PET-MR.

This article describes the application of various PET imaging agents in the investigation and diagnosis of Alzheimer's disease (AD), including radiotracers for pathologic biomarkers of AD such as β-amyloid deposits and tau protein aggregates, and the neuroinflammation biomarker 18 kDa translocator protein, as well as physiologic biomarkers, such as cholinergic receptors, glucose metabolism, and the synaptic density biomarker synaptic vesicle glycoprotein 2A. Potential of these biomarkers for early AD diagnosis is also assessed.

Biomarkers of the molecular pathology underpinning dementia syndromes are increasingly recognized as crucial for diagnosis and development of disease-modifying treatments. Amyloid PET imaging is an integral part of the diagnostic assessment of Alzheimer disease. Its use has also deepened understanding of the role of amyloid pathology in Lewy body disorders and aging. Tau PET imaging is an imaging biomarker that will likely play an important role in the diagnosis, monitoring, and treatment in dementias. Using tau PET imaging to examine how tau pathology relates to amyloid and other markers of neurodegeneration will serve to better understand the pathophysiologic cascade that leads to dementia.

As a result of high prevalence and high rates of treatment resistance, major depressive disorder has become the leading cause of death and disability in moderate-income to high-income nations. Poor targeting of phenotypes is a plausible reason for treatment resistance and PET imaging offers a unique role to identify phenotypes. Both increased monoamine oxidase A binding and greater translocator protein 18 kDa binding occur throughout the gray matter during major depressive episodes, including affect-modulating brain regions such as the prefrontal and anterior cingulate cortex, and are detectable with advanced radioligand technology for both of these targets.

PET CLINICS

RELATED INTEREST

Magnetic Resonance Imaging Clinics of North America,
May 2017 (Vol. 25, Issue 2)
Hybrid PET/MR Imaging
Weili Lin, Sheng-Che Hung, Yueh Z. Lee, and Terence Z. Wong, *Editors*
Available at: http://www.mri.theclinics.com/

THE CLINICS ARE AVAILABLE ONLINE!
Access your subscription at:
www.theclinics.com

PROGRAM OBJECTIVE
The goal of the *PET Clinics* is to keep practicing radiologists and radiology residents up to date with current clinical practice in positron emission tomography by providing timely articles reviewing the state of the art in patient care.

TARGET AUDIENCE
Practicing radiologists, radiology residents, and other healthcare professionals who provide patient care utilizing radiologic findings.

LEARNING OBJECTIVES
Upon completion of this activity, participants will be able to:
1. Review updates in radiotracer use for tumor treatment and prognosis.
2. Discuss the role of radiotracers in PET imaging for neurological conditions.
3. Recognize innovations in radiotracer use in PET-MR imaging.

ACCREDITATION
The Elsevier Office of Continuing Medical Education (EOCME) is accredited by the Accreditation Council for Continuing Medical Education (ACCME) to provide continuing medical education for physicians.

The EOCME designates this enduring material for a maximum of 15 *AMA PRA Category 1 Credit*(s)™. Physicians should claim only the credit commensurate with the extent of their participation in the activity.

All other healthcare professionals requesting continuing education credit for this enduring material will be issued a certificate of participation.

DISCLOSURE OF CONFLICTS OF INTEREST
The EOCME assesses conflict of interest with its instructors, faculty, planners, and other individuals who are in a position to control the content of CME activities. All relevant conflicts of interest that are identified are thoroughly vetted by EOCME for fair balance, scientific objectivity, and patient care recommendations. EOCME is committed to providing its learners with CME activities that promote improvements or quality in healthcare and not a specific proprietary business or a commercial interest.

The planning committee, staff, authors and editors listed below have identified no financial relationships or relationships to products or devices they or their spouse/life partner have with commercial interest related to the content of this CME activity:
Abass Alavi, MD, MD (Hon), PhD (Hon), DSc (Hon); Weiqi Bao, MD, PhD; Richard P. Baum, Prof, MD, PhD; Zhengxin Cai, PhD; Richard E. Carson, PhD; Georges El Fakhri, PhD; Sjoerd Finnema, PhD; Anjali Fortna; Kelly E. Henry, PhD; Yiyun Henry Huang, PhD; Hongmei Jia, PhD; Harshad Kulkarni, MD; Jason S. Lewis, PhD; Jeffrey Meyer, MD, PhD, FRCP(C); Yothin Rakvongthai, PhD; Steven P. Rowe, MD, PhD; Aviral Singh, MD; Gary A. Ulaner, MD, PhD; Neil Vasdev, PhD; John Vassallo; Rajakumar Venkatesan; Katie Widmeier; Amy Williams; Chenjie Xia, MD.

The planning committee, staff, authors and editors listed below have identified financial relationships or relationships to products or devices they or their spouse/life partner have with commercial interest related to the content of this CME activity:
Bradford C. Dickerson, MD is a consultant/advisor for Eli Lilly and Company.
Michael A. Gorin, MD is a consultant/advisor for, with research support from, Progenics Pharmaceuticals, Inc.
Andreas Kjaer, MD, PhD, DMSc is a co-founder at Curasight.
Theodosia Maina, PhD has research support from, and she and her spouse receive royalties/patents from, Advanced Accelerator Applications.
Berthold A. Nock, PhD and his spouse receive royalties/patents from, and his spouse has research support from, Advanced Accelerator Applications.
Morten Persson, MSc, PhD has stock ownership in Curasight.
Martin G. Pomper, MD, PhD has research support from, and receives royalties/patents from, Progenics Pharmaceuticals, Inc.
Dorthe Skovgaard, MD, PhD is a consultant/advisor for Curasight.

UNAPPROVED/OFF-LABEL USE DISCLOSURE
The EOCME requires CME faculty to disclose to the participants:
1. When products or procedures being discussed are off-label, unlabelled, experimental, and/or investigational (not US Food and Drug Administration [FDA] approved); and
2. Any limitations on the information presented, such as data that are preliminary or that represent ongoing research, interim analyses, and/or unsupported opinions. Faculty may discuss information about pharmaceutical agents that is outside of FDA-approved labelling. This information is intended solely for CME and is not intended to promote off-label use of these medications. If you have any questions, contact the medical affairs department of the manufacturer for the most recent prescribing information.

TO ENROLL

To enroll in the PET Clinics Continuing Medical Education program, call customer service at 1-800-654-2452 or sign up online at http://www.theclinics.com/home/cme. The CME program is available to subscribers for an additional annual fee of USD $235.

METHOD OF PARTICIPATION

In order to claim credit, participants must complete the following:

1. Complete enrolment as indicated above.
2. Read the activity.
3. Complete the CME Test and Evaluation. Participants must achieve a score of 70% on the test. All CME Tests and Evaluations must be completed online.

CME INQUIRIES/SPECIAL NEEDS

For all CME inquiries or special needs, please contact elsevierCME@elsevier.com.

Preface

Novel PET Radiotracers with Potential Clinical Applications

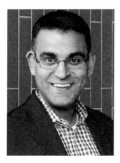
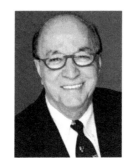

Neil Vasdev, PhD   Abass Alavi, MD, MD (Hon), PhD (Hon), DSc (Hon)

Editors

Since the introduction of radiopharmaceuticals for molecular imaging with PET, a great deal of effort has been made to expand the domain of this novel technology by discovery of specific labeled compounds to probe a variety of disorders. Significant advances have been made over the past four decades in generating PET images with high resolution and in great detail. While the original tomographic scanners designed and built in the 1970s and 1980s provided images with spatial resolution of 1 cm or higher, modern PET scanners have been designed to provide superb spatial resolutions in the range of several millimeters in humans. This has been achieved by increasing the number of detectors and developing sophisticated reconstruction algorithms that have overcome many of the shortcomings of the earlier-generation PET scanners. This trend has been particularly successful in preclinical and clinical imaging, where highly detailed images can be provided by modern instruments. Despite such advances made in PET instrumentation over the past two decades, PET is still considered to be a gross imaging modality, and therefore, it will fail in portraying details at the cellular and molecular levels if the intended tracer is not taken up by a target of relatively large mass. As such, extrapolating what is achieved in the in vitro testing of various compounds as well as on the autoradiographic images to human imaging is often overly simplistic. In order to image a biological phenomenon in normal and disease states, a large mass of cells (or other targets) needs to be localized in a volume that exceeds several cubic millimeters (realistically more than 1 cm^3) to be visualized by PET imaging. Furthermore, the degree of radiotracer uptake in such volumes has to be substantial and exceed the background activity at least by two to three times in order to achieve an acceptable contrast. With exciting scientific advances in instrumentation, pharmaceutical interests in applying PET in drug discovery, and novel radiochemistry methodologies, radiotracer development and preclinical PET imaging studies are at an all-time high. However, despite thousands of PET-labeled compounds and radiopharmaceuticals that have been reported in the literature over the past four decades, only a very small percentage of those have been translated for human use and less than 10 are approved PET radiopharmaceuticals by the US Food and Drug Administration. It is time to reevaluate our present-day strategies for radiopharmaceutical design and use in order to unveil the full potential of PET to deliver clinically relevant information on disease dynamics that extends beyond mapping the density and spatial distribution of a target.

The future of clinical applications of PET will depend on the next generation of rigorously designed and characterized radiopharmaceuticals, which specifically probe biological targets of interest in order to realize the full potential of "molecular imaging" as an evolving discipline in twenty-first century. It is our expectation that

http://dx.doi.org/10.1016/j.cpet.2017.04.002
1556-8598/17/© 2017 Published by Elsevier Inc.

this powerful approach will surpass competing imaging modalities in its impact on the day-to-day practice of medicine while being cost-effective. Recent developments in targeting pharmacodynamic biomarkers aim to further exploit the advantages of molecular imaging with PET by detecting changes in unexploited receptors, enzyme targets, and signal transduction pathways, specifically, in response to therapeutic interventions or disease progression. In this issue of *PET Clinics*, a selection of cutting-edge PET radiopharmaceuticals that have relatively recently been translated for imaging applications in human patient populations are highlighted. Particularly, we have emphasized their anticipated potential for widespread use and long-term clinical impact in a variety of diseases and disorders related to the subspecialties of oncology, cardiology, and neurology.

Neil Vasdev, PhD
Director of Radiochemistry
Massachusetts General Hospital
Associate Professor of Radiology
Division of Nuclear Medicine
and Molecular Imaging
Harvard Medical School
55 Fruit Street, White 427
Boston, MA 02114, USA

Abass Alavi, MD, MD (Hon), PhD (Hon), DSc (Hon)
Professor of Radiology and Neurology
Department of Radiology
Hospital of the University of Pennsylvania
3400 Spruce Street
Philadelphia, PA 19104, USA

E-mail addresses:
vasdev.neil@mgh.harvard.edu (N. Vasdev)
abass.alavi@uphs.upenn.edu (A. Alavi)

Human Epidermal Growth Factor Receptor 2-Targeted PET/Single-Photon Emission Computed Tomography Imaging of Breast Cancer

Noninvasive Measurement of a Biomarker Integral to Tumor Treatment and Prognosis

Kelly E. Henry, PhD[a],*, Gary A. Ulaner, MD, PhD[a,b],
Jason S. Lewis, PhD[a,c]

KEYWORDS

• PET • SPECT • CT • Imaging • Radiotracers • HER2 • Metastasis • Breast cancer

KEY POINTS

- Knowledge of the receptor status of breast cancer is integral to patient treatment and prognosis.
- Expression of estrogen receptor, progesterone receptor, and human epidermal growth factor receptor 2 (HER2) is assessed using immunohistochemistry, fluorescence in situ hybridization, or chromogen in situ hybridization.
- HER2 is expressed in low levels on the surface of normal cells but overexpressed in invasive breast cancers, a biomarker for aggressive breast cancer and response to HER2-targeted therapies.
- Monoclonal antibodies are used as HER2-targeted therapies, which can be labeled with positron-, gamma-emitting radionuclides for PET/computed tomography and single-photon emission computed tomography molecular imaging agents.
- PET imaging allows for noninvasive whole body analysis of tumors and may detect previously unsuspected HER2-positive metastases in patients with a HER2-negative primary breast tumor.

INTRODUCTION

Breast cancer is a heterogeneous disease in which tumor differentiation within lesions and in primary versus metastatic disease can be the basis of a poor prognosis and clinical outcomes.[1] Initial staging of breast cancer integrates pathologic analysis of receptor status in biopsied tissues. The three main biomarkers of interest in breast cancer include estrogen receptor (ER), progesterone

Disclosure Statement: The authors have nothing to disclose.
[a] Department of Radiology, Memorial Sloan Kettering Cancer Center, New York, NY 10065, USA;
[b] Department of Radiology, Weill Cornell Medical College, New York, NY 10065, USA; [c] Program in Molecular Pharmacology and Chemistry, Memorial Sloan Kettering Cancer Center, New York, NY 10065, USA
* Corresponding author. Department of Radiology, Memorial Sloan Kettering Cancer Center, 1275 York Avenue, New York, NY 10065.
E-mail address: henryk1@mskcc.org

receptor, and human epidermal growth factor receptor 2 (HER2).[2] These receptors are assessed using immunohistochemistry, fluorescence in situ hybridization, or chromogen in situ hybridization to direct therapy.[3]

HER2 overexpression is a hallmark of aggressive breast cancer, and its expression in a primary tumor directly influences treatment.[4] Because of this, HER2 has become a critical target for molecular imaging and therapy.[4,5] Approximately 20% of invasive ductal breast malignancies are classified as HER2 positive as a result of gene amplification and/or the subsequent overexpression of the HER2 protein on the surface of tumor cells.[6] Patients with HER2-positive breast cancer receive specific, targeted HER2 therapies to reduce the risk of death.[7] However, the current methods in the clinic to assess receptor status have issues when it comes to staging breast cancer, and consequently assigning therapy. Inherent errors include bias in and misinterpretation of immunohistochemistry or in situ hybridization results, sampling issues, and discordance between primary metastatic sites of disease.[8–10] Although not typically within the standard course of treatment, there have been reports of clinical benefit of HER2-targeted therapy even in patients with a primary HER2-negative tumor.[11] The hypothesis behind this phenomenon is owing to the heterogeneity of not just the primary tumors, but of metastatic disease as well.[12]

One approach to address these issues with current staging methods in HER2-positive breast cancer is to use targeted molecular imaging. Imaging modalities that target HER2 have the potential to not only diagnose HER2-positive breast cancer, but also detect distant metastases via a single, noninvasive procedure.[5,13,14] Molecular imaging, particularly with tracers used in PET, can address issues of heterogeneity and discordance between primary and metastatic disease in breast cancer. PET is especially useful when paired with methods for anatomic imaging (eg, MR imaging or computed tomography [CT]). These modalities used in tandem can detect exact location of disease, and allow more accurate surgical resection. PET imaging can also be used to select patients for targeted therapies and monitor treatment effects.[15]

PET is a highly sensitive, quantitative molecular imaging technique with high spatial resolution. PET is the select modality for imaging in the clinic owing to its favorable properties. Several groups have developed antibody-based radioligands over the past 15 years for PET imaging preclinically and clinically.[16–19] From this body of work, many of these targeted probes have been used to image HER2-positive breast cancer.[5,13] The clinical translation of antibodies has its drawbacks owing to often low tumor penetration because of high molecular weight (approximately 150 kDa) and slow clearance.[16] Also, conventional positron emitters (eg, ^{11}C, ^{13}N, ^{15}O, and ^{18}F) have half-lives that may be too short to permit adequate biodistribution of labeled antibodies before imaging. Pairing these targeting moieties with longer-lived radioisotopes such at zirconium-89 (^{89}Zr) for PET and indium-111 (^{111}In) for single-photon emission CT (SPECT) (^{89}Zr, $t_{1/2}$ = 78 hours; ^{111}In, $t_{1/2}$ = 67 hours) can be used to match the biological half-life of antibodies in vivo ($t_{1/2}$ approximately 72 hours), and allow radioactivity accumulation in tumors for up to 6 days.[20] Antibody fragments and affibody molecules (small proteins engineered to bind to a large number of target proteins or peptides with high affinity) can be labeled with shorter-lived isotopes such as gallium-68 (^{68}Ga) or fluorine-18 (^{18}F) (^{68}Ga, $t_{1/2}$ = 68 minutes; ^{18}F, $t_{1/2}$ = 110 minutes) for a faster turnaround and more transient detection of disease.[21–24] Isotopes with "medium" half-lives such as copper-64 (^{64}Cu, $t_{1/2}$ = 12 hours) are also used for both full-length and antibody fragments for PET imaging.[25–27]

Many of the PET and SPECT imaging tracers that have made it to the clinic (either in current clinical use, or have made it to phase I/II trials) to detect HER2-positive breast cancer and metastases, are summarized in **Table 1**. These agents are used for a more accurate diagnosis and patient selection for therapy in breast cancer.

Inaccurate knowledge of receptor status in metastases owing to tumor heterogeneity and differentiation throughout cancer spreading may lead to suboptimal selection of patients for HER2-targeted therapy.[12,28,29] Data show that more than 10% of patients with HER2-negative primary breast cancer may still benefit from HER2-targeted treatment.[11] This observation indicates that HER2-negative patients may have distant disease that is in fact HER2 positive. Targeting these metastases can reduce the risk of death in this aggressive subtype of breast cancer. Current treatments targeted to HER2-positive breast lesions, including hormone therapy, are listed in **Table 2**.

Trastuzumab is a monoclonal antibody that targets HER2 and is the first-line therapy for HER2-positive breast tumors.[29–32] The history of trastuzumab dates back to 1998 when it was approved by the Food and Drug Administration, and has been used regularly in the clinic ever since.[31] Imaging modalities have been constructed using a functionalized version of this antibody to detect HER2-positive disease and metastasis.

Table 1
Summary of clinical trials with PET and SPECT radiotracers targeting HER2-positive breast cancer

Radiotracer	Description of Trial	Clinical Trial or Reference	Sponsor	Status
[89]Zr-DFO-trastuzumab	HER2+ BC	NCT01832051	University Medical Center Groningen	Completed
	Imaging the effect of HSP90 inhibition	NCT01081600	University Medical Center Groningen	Completed
	HER2+ MBC	NCT01420146	Jules Bordet Institute	Completed
	HER2+ BC	NCT02065609	Washington University School of Medicine	Recruiting
	HER2+ MBC	NCT02286843	Memorial Sloan Kettering Cancer Center	Recruiting
	IMPACT-MBC	NCT01957332	University Medical Center Groningen	Recruiting
[64]Cu-DOTA-trastuzumab	HER2+ MBC	NCT00605397	Memorial Sloan Kettering Cancer Center	Completed
	Predicting treatment response in HER2+ BC	NCT02827877	City of Hope Medical Center	Verified
^{111}In-CHX-A DTPA-trastuzumab	HER2+ BC	NCT01445054	National Cancer Institute	Completed
[111]In-MxDTPA-trastuzumab	HER2+ BC	Wong et al,[49] 2010	City of Hope Medical Center	Completed
	HER2+ MBC	Perik et al,[47] 2006	University Medical Center Groningen	Completed
	HER2+ MBC	Gaykema et al,[48] 2014	University Medical Center Groningen	Completed
[68]Ga-F(ab')2-trastuzumab	HER2+ BC	NCT00613847	Memorial Sloan Kettering Cancer Center	Completed
^{68}Ga-ABY-025	HER2+ BC	NCT01858116	Biomedical Radiation Sciences	Completed
	HER2+ BC	NCT02095210	Dorte Nielsen	Recruiting
^{111}In-ABY-025	HER2+ MBC	NCT01216033	Biomedical Radiation Sciences	Completed
[64]Cu-MM-302	HER2+ MBC	NCT02735798	University of California, San Francisco	Verified
[^{131}I]-SGMIB anti-HER2 VHH1	Healthy Patients and HER2+ BC	NCT02683083	Camel-IDS NV	Recruiting
^{68}Ga-HER2-Nanobody	HER2+ BC	EudraCT 2012-001135-31	Vrije Universiteit Brussels	Completed

Abbreviations: BC, breast cancer; HER2, human epidermal growth factor 2; IMPACT, IMaging PAtients for Cancer Drug selecTion; MBC, metastatic breast cancer; SGMIB, N-succinimidyl 4-guanidinomethyl 3-iodobenzoate; SPECT, single photon emission computed tomography.

PET AND SINGLE PHOTON EMISSION COMPUTED TOMOGRAPHY IMAGING WITH MONOCLONAL ANTIBODIES IN HUMAN EPIDERMAL GROWTH FACTOR RECEPTOR 2-POSITIVE BREAST CANCER
Zirconium-89-DFO-Trastuzumab

[89]Zr radiopharmaceuticals are an attractive option for antibody-based imaging agents owing to their compatible half-life (approximately 78 hours) to monoclonal antibodies (approximately 72 hours).[20] Dijkers and colleagues[33] were the first to label clinical-grade trastuzumab with [89]Zr and use it for immunoPET imaging in animals. This radiotracer was later implemented to gauge HER2 status in not just primary tumor, but in patients with nonaccessible metastases.[33] With this product, Oude and colleagues[34] used [89]Zr-DFO-trastuzumab to annotate response of HER2 to HSP90 therapy preclinically. From here, there have been

Table 2
Drugs approved for anti-HER2 therapy in HER2-positive breast cancer

Drug (Chemical Name)	Classification	Mechanism of Action	Company	FDA Approved
Trastuzumab	Antibody	Binds to extracellular segment of the HER2/neu receptor	Genentech	1998
Pertuzumab	Antibody	Inhibits the dimerization of HER2 with other HER receptors	Genentech	2012
Ado-trastuzumab emtansine	Antibody–drug conjugate	Binds at plus ends of cellular microtubules and inhibits cell division in tumor cells	Genentech	2013
Lapatinib	Tyrosine kinase inhibitor	Interrupts HER2/neu and EGFR pathway	GlaxoSmithKline	2007

Abbreviations: EGFR, epidermal growth factor receptor; FDA, Food and Drug Administration; HER2, human epidermal growth factor 2.

numerous reports of preclinical and clinical studies with this tracer that have evolved both imaging and therapy within HER2-positive breast cancer.

[89]Zr-DFO-trastuzumab has been favored owing to a higher spatial resolution and a better signal-to-noise ratio than ^{111}In-trastuzumab, and ease of data quantification with PET versus SPECT. Preliminary results (Dijkers and colleagues[35]) with [89]Zr-DFO-trastuzumab immunoPET in HER2-positive breast cancer patients indicated exceptional tumor uptake and spatial resolution. Fourteen patients with HER2-positive metastatic breast cancer received 37 MBq of [89]Zr-trastuzumab at 1 of 3 doses (10 or 50 mg for those who had not received trastuzumab and 10 mg for those who were undergoing trastuzumab treatment). The patients underwent serial PET scans between days 2 and 5. The results of the study showed that the best time for assessment of the uptake of [89]Zr-trastuzumab was 4 to 5 days after injection. **Fig. 1** represents the biodistribution of [89]Zr-DFO-trastuzumab, including detection of metastatic brain lesions that were not observed by fludeoxyglucose F 18 (^{18}F-FDG). Fusion PET/MR imaging

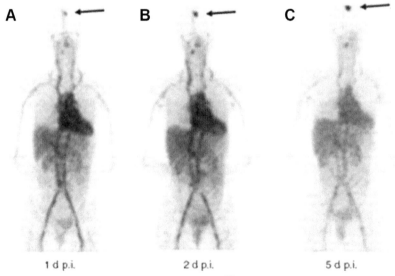

A   B   C

1 d p.i.   2 d p.i.   5 d p.i.

Fig. 1. [89]Zr-trastuzumab biodistribution in time. (*A–C*) Three [89]Zr-trastuzumab scans of a patient already on trastuzumab treatment (cohort 3) show the increase over time in the tumor/nontumor ratio with regard to uptake of the tracer. Arrow indicates [89]Zr-trastuzumab uptake in the only lesion. p.i., postinjection; [89]Zr, zirconium-89. (*From* Dijkers EC, Oude Munnink TH, Kosterink JG, et al. Biodistribution of 89Zr-trastuzumab and PET imaging of HER2-positive lesions in patients with metastatic breast cancer. Clin Pharmacol Ther 2010;87(5):588; with permission.)

scans in **Fig. 2** further highlight this observation, revealing the true usefulness of this radiotracer in patients. This pilot study showed promise in the ability of [89]Zr-DFO-trastuzumab to detect not only primary tumor, but also metastatic disease that conventional PET was unable to accomplish.[36]

Zirconium-89-DFO-Trastuzumab to Detect Unsuspected Human Epidermal Growth Factor Receptor 2-Positive Metastatic Disease

Ulaner and colleagues[12] explored the potential of [89]Zr-DFO-trastuzumab to detect HER2-positive metastases in HER2-negative primary tumors. Nine patients with HER2-negative primary breast

A　　　　　　　　　　**B**

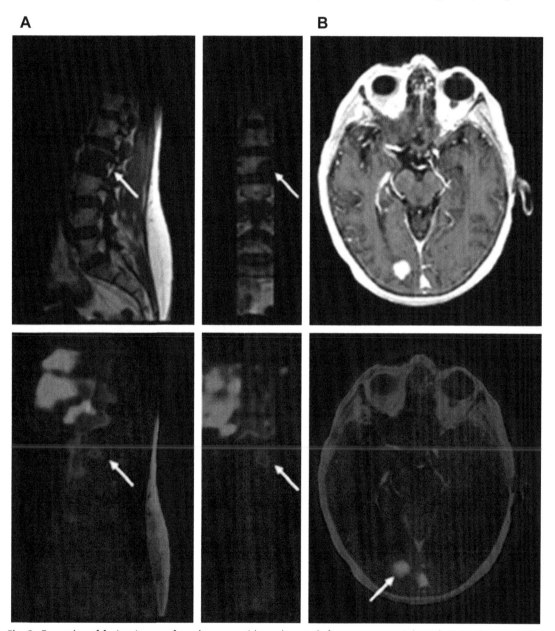

Fig. 2. Examples of fusion images from human epidermal growth factor receptor 2 (HER2) PET and MR imaging scans. (A) In a vertebral metastasis seen on MR imaging but unapproachable for biopsy, HER2 status was revealed by [89]Zr-trastuzumab uptake on PET imaging. (B) Example of HER2-positive brain lesion undetected by conventional scans, revealed by [89]Zr-trastuzumab PET imaging, and subsequently confirmed by MR imaging. Arrows indicate lesions. HER2, human epidermal growth factor receptor 2; [89]Zr, zirconium-89. (From Dijkers EC, Oude Munnink TH, Kosterink JG, et al. Biodistribution of 89Zr-trastuzumab and PET imaging of HER2-positive lesions in patients with metastatic breast cancer. Clin Pharmacol Ther 2010;87(5):589; with permission.)

cancer were enrolled in this study, and imaged with [89]Zr-DFO-trastuzumab PET/CT to detect for [89]Zr-DFO-trastuzumab–avid metastases. All patients enrolled were confirmed pathologically as HER2 negative. Metastases that were observed via [89]Zr-trastuzumab PET/CT were biopsied and pathologically examined to define HER2 status. Based on these findings, patients with HER2-positive metastases received HER2-targeted therapy to evaluate treatment response. An example of one such patient is represented in **Fig. 3**.

Of the 9 patients, 5 exhibited metastatic uptake with [89]Zr-DFO-trastuzumab PET/CT. Of these 5 patients, 2 had biopsies taken of potential metastatic sites based from their PET scans. These 2 patients exhibited HER2-positive metastases (as confirmed via pathologic workup of the biopsied tissue) and subsequently benefitted from HER2-targeted therapy. The remaining 3 patients with suspicious uptake were also biopsied, and did not present evidence of HER2-positive disease at metastatic lesions, and were considered false positive for [89]Zr-DFO-trastuzumab PET. An example of a false-positive scan is presented in **Fig. 4**.[12]

The significant result of this study is that [89]Zr-DFO-trastuzumab PET/CT can detect unsuspected HER2-positive metastases in patients with a HER2-negative primary breast cancer. Although these preliminary results encompass a small sample size, it still gives strong evidence that HER2-targeted imaging can identify candidates for HER2-targeted therapy. These results provide a possible explanation for the hypothesis that a minority of patients with HER2-negative tumors benefit from HER2-targeted therapy because of the heterogeneity within distant disease. More specific HER2-targeting agents are necessary in the clinic to elucidate fully this relationship via imaging, and decrease the potential for false-positive uptake.

Annotating Treatment Response with Zirconium-89-DFO-Trastuzumab

Heath shock protein 90 (HSP90) is an ATP-dependent molecular chaperone protein that is involved in several oncogenic pathways, and has been a target for many cancer therapies.[37] HSP90 inhibitors have emerged as a promising anticancer strategy in many cancers, including HER2-positive breast cancer.[38] HSP90 inhibitors have been combined with trastuzumab (either as

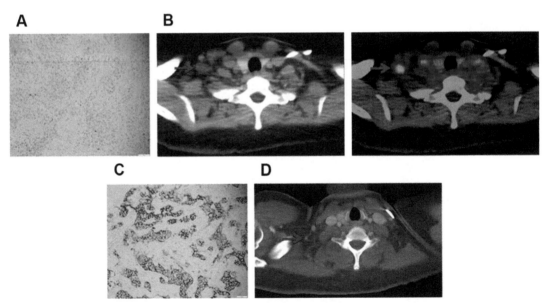

Fig. 3. A 41-year-old woman with primary ER-positive, human epidermal growth factor receptor 2 (HER2)-negative invasive ductal breast carcinoma and recurrence in the thoracic nodes. (*A*) Immunohistochemistry score of primary breast malignancy was 11 (at 20× magnification), consistent with HER2-negative malignancy. (*B*) Axial computed tomography (CT) and [89]Zr-trastuzumab PET/CT demonstrated [89]Zr-trastuzumab avidity in enlarged right supraclavicular nodes (*arrows*, maximum standardized uptake value of 4.6) and left internal mammary nodes (not shown). (*C*) Biopsy of right supraclavicular node demonstrated metastatic breast carcinoma with immunohistochemistry score of 31 (at 20× magnification), consistent with HER2-positive disease. The patient began systemic treatment including trastuzumab and pertuzumab. (*D*) Follow-up axial CT after 2 months of treatment demonstrated resolution of nodes on CT examination (*arrow*). (*From* Ulaner GA, Hyman DM, Ross DS, et al. Detection of HER2-positive metastases in patients with HER2-negative primary breast cancer using 89Zr-trastuzumab PET/CT. J Nuc Med 2016;57(10):1526; with permission.)

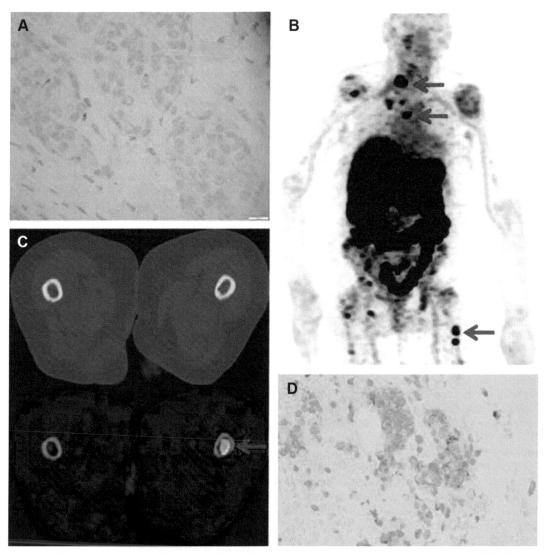

Fig. 4. An 83-year-old woman with primary ER-positive/human epidermal growth factor receptor 2 (HER2)-negative invasive ductal breast carcinoma. (*A*) Immunohistochemistry score of primary breast malignancy was 11 (at 400× magnification), consistent with HER2-negative malignancy. (*B*) ^{89}Zr-trastuzumab maximum intensity projection demonstrates several foci of ^{89}Zr-trastuzumab avidity that localize to osseous structures (*arrows*). Avidity in liver and bowel is considered physiologic. (*C*) Axial computed tomography (CT) and ^{89}Zr-trastuzumab PET/CT demonstrate ^{89}Zr-trastuzumab avidity in proximal left femur (*arrow*; maximum standardized uptake value of 7.7). (*D*) Biopsy of proximal left femur demonstrated metastatic breast carcinoma with immunohistochemistry score of 11 (at 400× magnification), consistent with HER2-negative disease. (*From* Ulaner GA, Hyman DM, Ross DS, et al. Detection of HER2-positive metastases in patients with HER2-negative primary breast cancer using 89Zr-trastuzumab PET/CT. J Nuc Med 2016;57(10):1527; with permission.)

treatment or assessing treatment response) in HER2-positive metastatic breast cancer.[39]

The primary aim of a clinical trial led by Gaykema and colleagues[34] was to evaluate the usefulness of ^{89}Zr-DFO-trastuzumab PET (for HER2-positive breast cancer) or ^{89}Zr-DFO-bevacizumab PET (for ER-positive breast cancer) to determine the in vivo degradation of proteins owing to HSP90 inhibitor NVP-AUY922. Sixteen patients (10 HER2-positive and 6 ER-positive tumors) were included in this study. During this study, NVP-AUY922 (70 mg/m^2) was administered intravenously weekly to patients with advanced HER2- or ER-positive breast cancer. Serial PET imaging with ^{18}F-FDG, ^{89}Zr-DFO-trastuzumab, or ^{89}Zr-DFO-bevacizumab was performed to assess biomarkers of interest (HER2, ER, and ^{18}F-FDG used as a metabolic marker). Blood samples were collected to detect HSP90 levels and the extracellular form of HER2. One partial response was observed from NVP-AUY922 treatment, and 7 patients showed no response. Changes in the maximum standardized uptake value in patients with [89]Zr-trastuzumab PET before and after treatment was heterogeneous and correlated with size change on CT. Treatment with HSP90 inhibitor NVP-AUY922 showed a clinical response in HER2-positive metastatic breast cancer. Changes in [89]Zr-DFO-trastuzumab PET were concomitant with change in size of lesions, as measured by CT.

Another ongoing study to assess the usefulness of [89]Zr-trastuzumab to image therapy response is the ZEPHIR trial (Phase II Prospective Imaging Study Evaluating the Utility of Pre-treatment Zr[89] Labelled Trastuzumab PET/CT and an Early FDG-PET/CT Response to Identify Patients With Advanced HER2+ BC Unlikely to Benefit From a Novel anti-HER2 Therapy: TDM1), led by the Jules Bordet Institute. This clinical trial is currently enrolling patients from Belgium and the Netherlands eligible to receive that antibody–drug conjugate T-DM1 for HER2-positive advanced disease. HER2-positive metastatic breast cancer patients with an immunohistochemistry 3+ or a fluorescence in situ hybridization score of greater than 2.2 eligible for T-DM1 treatment underwent a pretreatment PET/CT scan with [89]Zr-trastuzumab. ^{18}F-FDG PET/CT was performed at baseline and before T-DM1 cycle 2. Patients were grouped into 4 HER2–PET/CT patterns according to the proportion of ^{18}F-FDG–avid tumor concurrent with [89]Zr-trastuzumab uptake. In the 56 patients analyzed, 29% had negative [89]Zr-trastuzumab PET/CT and intrapatient heterogeneity was found in 46% of patients.[40] [89]Zr-trastuzumab imaging, combined with early metabolic response assessment with ^{18}F-FDG accurately predicted morphologic response after 3 treatment cycles with T-DM1. This methodology has the potential for improving the understanding of tumor heterogeneity in metastatic breast cancer and for selecting patients who may or may not benefit from T-DM1.

Currently, patients are still being recruited for many [89]Zr-DFO-trastuzumab PET imaging trials. The IMPACT trial (IMaging PAtients for Cancer Drug selecTion) for metastatic breast cancer, led by the University Medical Center Groningen, is using [89]Zr-DFO-trastuzumab for baseline scans to recruit patients for antibody therapy.[41] Another trial has been completed at the Jules Bordet Institute to assess [89]Zr-DFO-trastuzumab uptake in metastatic breast cancer,[42] and the ZEPHIR trial is still recruiting patients to increase the number of patients that may potentially benefit from T-DM1 therapy.[43] Patients are still being recruited

at Memorial Sloan Kettering Cancer Center to extend the usefulness of [89]Zr-DFO-trastuzumab to detect metastatic disease in HER2-negative primary breast cancer.[44] The Washington University School of Medicine is recruiting patients headlining their own clinical trial to assess uptake and dosimetry of [89]Zr-DFO-trastuzumab in patients.[45] Overall, [89]Zr-DFO-trastuzumab is an extremely useful clinical tool for assessing HER2-positive breast cancer, and has proven useful as a method to detect heterogeneity within both primary and metastatic lesions. The future of this radiotracer lies in its capacity for patient selection, which is what the IMPACT trial and the Memorial Sloan Kettering Cancer Center study aim to accomplish.

Copper-64-DOTA-Trastuzumab

The transition to shorter-lived PET radioisotopes started with ^{64}Cu-labeling of trastuzumab. The first study was to determine the safety, distribution, internal dosimetry, and initial HER2-positive tumor images of ^{64}Cu-DOTA-trastuzumab in humans by Tamura and colleagues.[26] PET imaging was performed on 6 patients with primary or metastatic HER2-positive breast cancer at 1, 24, and 48 hours after injection of approximately 130 MBq of the tracer ^{64}Cu-DOTA-trastuzumab. Samples were collected from the blood, urine, and nontarget tissue samples to assess the biodistribution and internal dosimetry of the probe.[26] The results from this study identified 48 hours as the best time point for ^{64}Cu-DOTA-trastuzumab after injection (Fig. 5).

An important outcome from this study was identifying that the radiation exposure during ^{64}Cu-DOTA-trastuzumab PET was comparable with that during ^{18}F-FDG PET, which is the conventional tracer for PET imaging in the clinic. Although the radioactivity in the blood was high, the uptake of ^{64}Cu-DOTA-trastuzumab in nontarget tissues was low, which is critical for improving detection. Brain metastases were observed in 2 patients that were administered ^{64}Cu-DOTA-trastuzumab PET, indicative of blood–brain barrier passage of the antibody tracer (Fig. 6). In 3 patients, ^{64}Cu-DOTA-trastuzumab PET imaging also revealed primary breast tumors in areas that were initially identified by CT. The findings of this study indicated that ^{64}Cu-DOTA-trastuzumab PET could detect HER2-positive lesions in patients with both primary and metastatic breast cancer.

Copper-64-DOTA-Trastuzumab in Metastatic Disease

Owing to successful identification of brain metastasis from HER2-positive primary breast tumors, a more focused study was done by Kurihara and

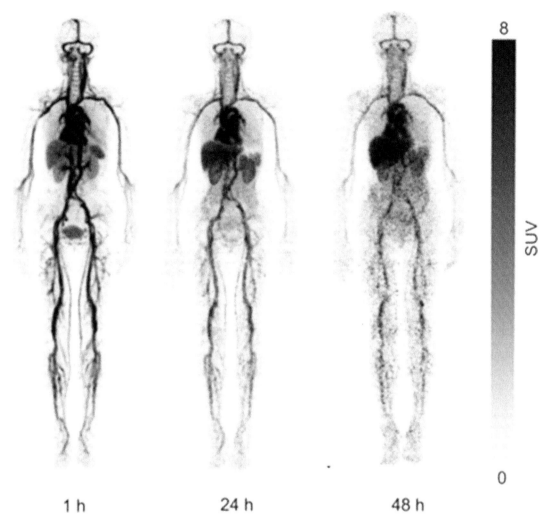

8

SUV

0

| 1 h | 24 h | 48 h |

Fig. 5. Whole-body copper-64-DOTA-trastuzumab PET images at 1, 24, and 48 hours after injection (patient 4). (*From* Tamura K, Kurihara H, Yonemori K, et al. 64Cu-DOTA-trastuzumab PET imaging in patients with HER2-positive breast cancer. J Nucl Med 2013;54(11):1871; with permission.)

colleagues[25] with ^{64}Cu-DOTA-trastuzumab PET in HER2-positive metastatic breast cancer. PET imaging was performed on 5 patients with confirmed brain metastases from HER2-positive breast cancer, at 24 or 48 hours after the injection of approximately 130 MBq of ^{64}Cu-DOTA-trastuzumab. ^{64}Cu-DOTA-trastuzumab PET visualized metastatic brain lesions in all 5 patients (**Fig. 7**). This study gave further evidence that trastuzumab may pass through the blood–brain barrier and is able to detect HER2-positive metastases. From these studies, ^{64}Cu-DOTA-trastuzumab PET could be a potential noninvasive procedure for serial identification of metastatic brain lesions in patients with HER2-positive breast cancer.[25]

In summary, ^{64}Cu-DOTA-trastuzumab has been successful in detecting both primary and

metastatic disease in patients. Currently, patients are being recruited at the City of Hope Medical Center to use ^{64}Cu-DOTA-trastuzumab to predict treatment response with trastuzumab and pertuzumab before surgery in HER2-positive breast cancer.[46] The future of this tracer will be assessed by this trial and its involvement in predicting treatment response and facilitating patient selection for antibody therapy in HER2-positive breast cancer.

Indium-111-Trastuzumab

Trastuzumab functionalized as an SPECT molecular imaging probe began with the pairing of the antibody to the SPECT isotope, indium-111 (^{111}In). ^{111}In-MxDTPA-trastuzumab imaging was done by Perik and colleagues[47] to assess effects

A

B   Axial   Coronal

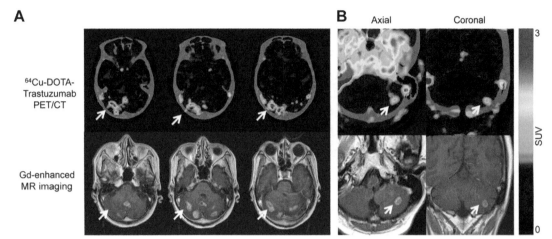

^{64}Cu-DOTA-
Trastuzumab
PET/CT

Gd-enhanced
MR imaging

Fig. 6. Copper-64 (^{64}Cu)-DOTA-trastuzumab PET images of human epidermal growth factor receptor 2 (HER2)-positive metastatic brain lesions (*arrows*). (*A*) Brain metastases were clearly visualized by ^{64}Cu-DOTA-trastuzumab PET in patient 1. Significant uptake values were found in areas corresponding to brain metastatic lesions that were detected by MR imaging. Some brain metastases could not be detected on conventional CT. (*B*) In patient 4, ^{64}Cu-DOTA-trastuzumab PET imaging could detect solitary brain metastasis that had also been identified in similar location by MR imaging. Gd, gadolinium. (*From* Tamura K, Kurihara H, Yonemori K, et al. 64Cu-DOTA-trastuzumab PET imaging in patients with HER2-positive breast cancer. J Nucl Med 2013;54(11):1874; with permission.)

and clinical benefit of trastuzumab therapy. The ultimate result from this study was to confirm that HER2 imaging is feasible during trastuzumab treatment, and can successfully annotate response. It was concluded that the same antibody could be used for both treatment and therapy benefit in the same patient. This was further confirmed in a follow-up study also done by Gaykema and colleagues,[48] who showed that treatment with trastuzumab in patients resulted in decreased tumor ^{111}In-MxDTPA-trastuzumab uptake of about 20%.

Wong and colleagues[49] evaluated the organ biodistribution, pharmacokinetics, immunogenicity,

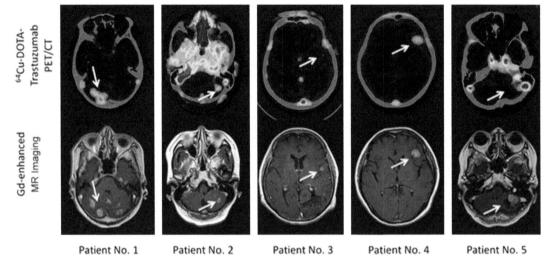

^{64}Cu-DOTA-
Trastuzumab
PET/CT

Gd-enhanced
MR Imaging

Patient No. 1   Patient No. 2   Patient No. 3   Patient No. 4   Patient No. 5

Fig. 7. Copper-64 (^{64}Cu)-DOTA-trastuzumab PET images of metastatic brain tumors in patients with human epidermal growth factor receptor 2 (HER2)-positive primary breast tumors. The white arrows show the metastatic brain tumors. Upper panels: ^{64}Cu-DOTA-trastuzumab PET images. Lower panels: gadolinium (Gd)-DTPA-enhanced T1-weighted MR imaging images. White arrows indicate metastatic brain lesions detectable by both MR imaging and ^{64}Cu-DOTA-trastuzumab PET, and the red arrow indicates a lesion detectable by MR imaging but not by ^{64}Cu-DOTA-trastuzumab PET. In the PET image from patient 2, nonspecific high uptake in the blood was noted. (*From* Kurihara H, Hamada A, Yoshida M, et al. 64Cu-DOTA-trastuzumab PET imaging and HER2 specificity of brain metastases in HER2-positive breast cancer patients. EJNMMI Res 2015;5(8):4; with permission.)

and tumor uptake of ^{111}In-MxDTPA-trastuzumab in patients with HER2-overexpressing breast cancers and to determine whether ^{90}Y-trastuzumab should be evaluated in subsequent clinical therapy trials. Patients with HER2-overexpressing breast cancers that were scheduled to receive trastuzumab therapy first underwent (unlabeled) trastuzumab therapy (4–8 mg/kg), followed by 185 MBq ^{111}In-MxDTPA-trastuzumab (10 mg, 4 hours after therapy). Blood and urine samples (24 hours) were obtained for further analysis. Nuclear scans were performed at defined time points for 7 days. Eight patients received ^{111}In-MxDTPA-trastuzumab, which was well-tolerated with no adverse side effects. Three of 7 patients with known lesions showed positive tracer uptake in PET imaging. No immunogenic responses were observed for 2 months after injection, indicating the safety of the tracer.

The outcome of this study indicates that ^{90}Y-trastuzumab may be an appropriate agent to evaluate further in the clinic. No immunogenic response to ^{111}In-MxDTPA-trastuzumab was observed, and the pharmacokinetics and organ biodistribution were comparable with other ^{90}Y-labeled monoclonal antibodies. Cardiac uptake was a slight concern/difference to other radioimmunotherapy antibodies in the clinic, but was found to be similar to hepatic uptake and not expected to cause dose-limiting cardiotoxicity. HER2-targeted therapy and subsequent interrogation of these treatment effects through imaging could be a useful tool for predicting patient response. This would allow physicians to identify patients that do and do not respond to targeted therapies, opening educated options of pursuing different avenues of treatment.

The National Cancer Institute also currently sponsors a clinical trial to assess the effects of ^{111}In-CHX-A DTPA-trastuzumab imaging in HER2-positive breast cancer. Fluorescence in situ hybridization at both primary and metastatic sites of breast cancer is used to assess HER2 status. The results of these studies have yet to be published.

Indium-111-DTPA-Pertuzumab

Pertuzumab is another monoclonal antibody marketed by Genentech for treatment for HER2-positive breast cancer.[50] This therapy is often used in tandem with trastuzumab and docetaxel.[51] Pertuzumab inhibits dimerization of HER2 with other HER2 receptors, which is thought to slow tumor growth.[50] A clinical trial was attempted to recruit patients with imaging with ^{111}In-DTPA-pertuzumab to predict response to trastuzumab in HER2-positive metastatic breast cancer, but this trial was terminated owing to poor accrual of patients.[52] [89]Zr-DFO-pertuzumab has also been explored preclinically,[53] but has not yet reached clinical trials, likely owing to the high interest and success with [89]Zr-DFO-trastuzumab.

Iodine-131-SGMID Anti-Her2 VHH1

A monoclonal antibody directed against HER2 (VHH1) labeled with iodine-131 (^{131}I) with the radio-iodinating reagent N-succinimidyl 4-guanidinomethyl 3-iodobenzoate (SGMIB), is also being explored in the clinic for potential imaging of HER2-positive breast cancer.[54] SGMIB improves internalization and subsequent tumor retention of radioactivity, which has potential to improve on the current state of antibody imaging. The primary goal of the aforementioned clinical trial is to evaluate the safety, biodistribution, and dosimetry of [^{131}I]-SGMIB anti-HER2 VHH1 in both healthy volunteers and patients with HER2-positive breast cancer. Tumor targeting potential of [^{131}I]-SGMIB anti-HER2 VHH1 in patients with HER2-positive breast cancer will also be explored in this clinical study.

Copper-64-MM-302

MM-302 is an antibody–drug conjugate of HER2-targeted liposomal doxorubicin, as a single therapy or in combination with trastuzumab or trastuzumab and cyclophosphamide, and is currently being explored in clinical trials.[55,56] Initial results showed that the drug was safe and efficacious in a group of pretreated women with HER2-positive metastatic breast cancer. MM-302 labeled with ^{64}Cu is currently being used as an imaging agent for patient selection for combination therapy with trastuzumab and MM-302 in HER2-positive metastatic cancer, including breast. Patients will receive standard imaging at baseline (^{18}F-FDG PET/CT), along with MR brain imaging. Patients will then receive ^{64}Cu-MM-302 after MM-302 administration, and continue to receive subsequent doses of unlabeled MM-302 plus trastuzumab every 3 weeks and to be assessed for disease progression.[57]

ANTIBODY FRAGMENTS IN CLINICAL PET IMAGING

^{68}Ga-DOTA-F(ab')2-trastuzumab has been developed at Memorial Sloan Kettering Cancer Center as a PET imaging reagent for assessing HER2 expression status by in vivo imaging.[58] Preclinical studies demonstrated promising results in the monitoring of treatment response to HSP90-targeted drugs that inhibit HER2.[59] Initial clinical data were collected to assess the toxicity,

pharmacokinetics, biodistribution, and dosimetry profile of ^{68}Ga-DOTA-F(ab')2-trastuzumab with PET/CT. Beylergil and colleagues[58] led this study, where 16 women with breast cancer were enrolled in this clinical trial, with 1 patient who did not receive ^{68}Ga-DOTA-F(ab')2-trastuzumab and was excluded from analysis. HER2-negative (n = 7) and HER2-positive (n = 8) cases were studied in this initial study. In the HER2-positive group, 7 had received trastuzumab treatment previously and 1 had not. It was determined that ^{68}Ga-DOTA-F(ab')2-trastuzumab was well-tolerated, and tumor targeting was seen in 4 of the 8 patients with HER2-positive disease. Serial imaging of a single patient is represented in **Fig. 8**. ^{68}Ga-DOTA-F(ab')2-trastuzumab was also successful in detecting metastatic disease (**Figs. 9** and **10**). It was hypothesized that high circulating levels of trastuzumab inhibiting with tumor targeting by ^{68}Ga-DOTA-F(ab')2-trastuzumab, and could explain only 50% of targeting of known (^{18}F-FDG confirmed) lesions.

CLINICAL PET IMAGING WITH RADIOLABELED AFFIBODIES
Indium-111-ABY-025 and Gallium-68-ABY-025

Affibody molecules are small affinity ligands that are designed to mimic antibody-binding properties.[60] Affibodies are capable of binding to a wide range of protein targets and are used for diagnostic imaging and therapy applications. The

first clinical studies using radiolabeled affibodies were performed by Baum and colleagues,[23] with ^{111}In- or ^{68}Ga-labeled ABY-002 for imaging HER2-expressing malignant breast tumors. Three patients with metastatic breast cancer and known lesions (as identified by CT and/or ^{18}F-FDG PET/CT) received approximately 80 to 90 µg of radiolabeled ABY-002. Two patients received both ^{111}In-ABY-002 and ^{68}Ga-ABY-002, and 1 patient received ^{68}Ga-ABY-002 only. Rapid blood clearance of radiolabeled ABY-002 was observed and allowed for quality images with both SPECT and PET radionuclides as quickly as 2 hours after injection. Radiolabeled ABY-002 was detected in metastatic lesions, along with background uptake in the kidneys and the liver. The majority of identified lesions (via ^{18}F-FDG PET) were successfully observed using ABY-002 imaging. However, 2 sites of metastatic lesions (near the kidney and liver) were positive on ^{18}F-FDG PET/CT scans, but not observed with ABY-002 imaging, owing to high background accumulation in these organs.[61] Therefore, these particular tracers were not pursued further, but the affibodies were modified to improve background radioactivity and clearance of the ligand. The benefit of affibodies in molecular imaging is the fast pharmacokinetics and overall turnaround, but further clinical studies are required to optimize the dose, time, sensitivity, and specificity of these ligands.

Another version of affibody molecule for HER2-targeted imaging (ABY-025) was developed by

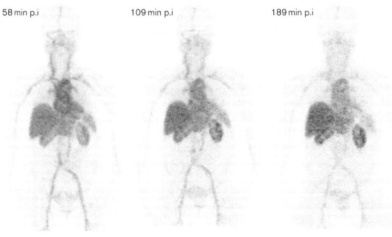

Fig. 8. Serial MIP images (patient 6) displayed at the same relative intensity. Although a slight decrease in blood pool is present, blood pool activity dominates the distribution. At 58, 109, and 189 minutes, the blood pool has a maximum standardized uptake value of 16.9, 13.6, and 9.8, respectively. There is slight increased uptake over time in the liver and kidneys. The patient had human epidermal growth factor 2 (HER2)-positive disease and was receiving lapatinib. Tumors in the left adrenal, hilar nodes, and bones were not visualized on Ga-PET. HER2, human epidermal growth factor receptor 2; MIP, maximum intensity projection; p.i, postinjection. (*From* Beyergil V, Morris PG, Smith-Jones PM, et al. Pilot study of 68Ga-DOTA-F(ab')2-trastuzumab in patients with breast cancer. Nucl Med Commun 2013;34(12):1162; with permission.)

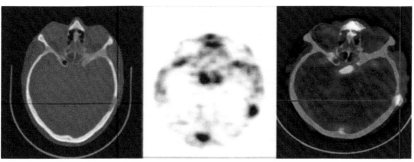

Fig. 9. Lytic lesion in the left calvarium with gallium-68 (^{68}Ga)-DOTA-F(ab')2-trastuzumab uptake (patient 1). ^{68}Ga-DOTA-F(ab')2-trastuzumab, ^{68}Ga-1,4,7,10-tetraazacyclododecane- N,N',N',N'''-tetraacetic acid (DOTA)-F(ab') 2-trastuzumab. (*From* Beyergil V, Morris PG, Smith-Jones PM, et al. Pilot study of 68Ga-DOTA-F(ab')2-trastuzumab in patients with breast cancer. Nucl Med Commun 2013;34(12):1163; with permission.)

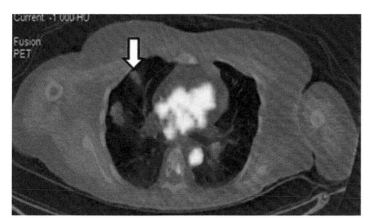

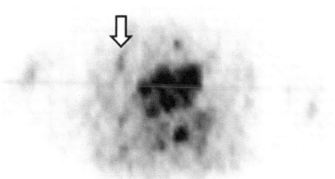

Fig. 10. In patient 2, fused images obtained at B1 hours show mild ^{68}Ga-DOTAF(ab')2-trastuzumab uptake in a lung metastasis (*arrows*). ^{68}Ga-DOTA-F(ab')2- trastuzumab, ^{68}Ga-1,4,7,10-tetraazacyclododecane-N,N',N',N'''-tetraacetic acid (DOTA)-F(ab')2-trastuzumab. (*From* Beyergil V, Morris PG, Smith-Jones PM, et al. Pilot study of 68Ga-DOTA-F(ab')2-trastuzumab in patients with breast cancer. Nucl Med Commun 2013; 34(12):1163; with permission.)

Fig. 11. Representative whole-body images at 10, 30, 60, 120, and 240 minutes after injection of a low and high peptide dose in the same patient. (*From* Sandström M, Lindskog K, Velikyan I, et al. Biodistribution and radiation dosimetry of the anti-HER2 affibody molecule 68Ga-ABY-025 in breast cancer patients. J Nuc Med 2016; 57(6):868; with permission.)

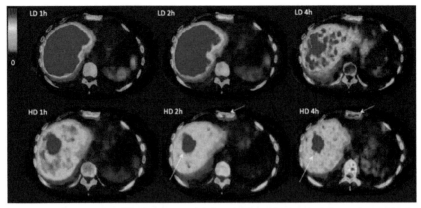

Fig. 12. Uptake images of gallium-68 (^{68}Ga)-BY-025 with low (LD) and high administered peptide dose (HD) at 1, 2 and 4 hours after injection in patient 2. All images are normalized to the same scale of standardized uptake value 10. A rainbow color scale is used: red color, standardized uptake value of greater than 10. Normal soft tissue uptake was higher with LD. Note the gradually higher contrast of metastases in liver and bone (*arrows*), owing to both the disappearance of normal liver uptake and tumor uptake accumulation. (*From* Sörensen J, Velikyan I, Sandberg D, et al. Measuring HER2-receptor expression in metastatic breast cancer using [68Ga]ABY-025 affibody PET/CT. Theranostics 2016;6(2):266; with permission.)

Sörensen and colleagues[22] ABY-025 is a reengineered affibody molecule that targets an exclusive epitope of the HER2 receptor that is not targeted by other HER2-targeted therapeutics. The advance of ABY-025 (vs ABY-002) lies in the improved tumor/background ratios, allowing for successful detection metastatic disease (most importantly in the liver) to be observed. A preliminary study

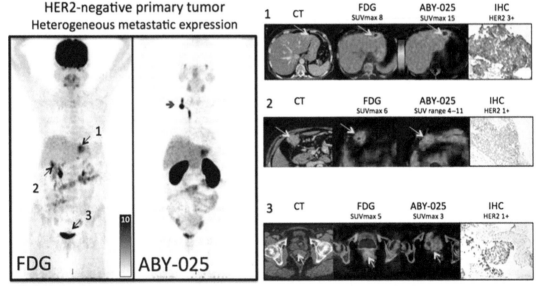

➜ Portacath used for injection

Fig. 13. Based on the results from gallium-68-ABY-025 PET/computed tomography (CT), mixed expression of human epidermal growth factor receptor 2 (HER2) in metastatic breast cancer was seen in several patients (*arrows*) and confirmed by biopsies in 2. Patient 9 had HER2-negative primary tumor and was enrolled as negative control. Fluorodeoxyglucose (FDG)-PET/CT showed metastases in left liver lobe, peritoneal lymph nodes and cervix of uterus (*arrows*). ABY-025 uptake was high in the liver metastasis, low in peritoneal metastases and absent in the cervical region (not shown). According to immunohistochemistry (IHC), the liver finding was true positive and both other sites were true negative. SUV$_{max}$, maximum standardized uptake volume. (*From* Sörensen J, Velikyan I, Sandberg D, et al. Measuring HER2-receptor expression in metastatic breast cancer using [68Ga] ABY-025 affibody PET/CT. Theranostics 2016;6(2):268; with permission.)

A

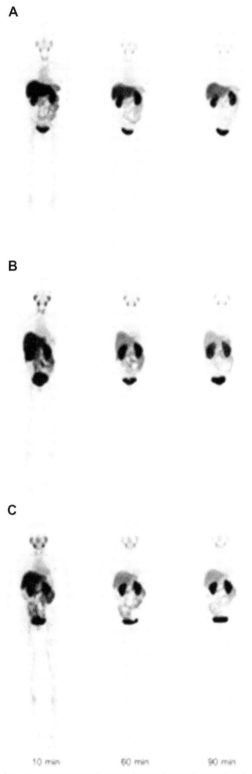

B

C

10 min   60 min   90 min

Fig. 14. Representative maximum intensity projection images at 10, 60, and 90 minutes after injection of gallium-68 (^{68}Ga)-human epidermal growth factor receptor 2 (HER2)-nanobody for different mass subgroups. (*A*) Patient 4, injected with 0.01 mg of

evaluated the biodistribution, safety, dosimetry, and tumor-targeting potential of ^{111}In-ABY-025 for assessing HER2 status in metastatic breast cancer. Seven patients with metastatic breast cancer and HER2-positive or negative primary tumors received approximately 100 μg (approximately 140 MBq) of ^{111}In-ABY-025. SPECT/CT imaging was performed after 4, 24, and 48 hours. Blood samples were taken to measure radioactivity, antibodies, serum HER2, and toxicity markers. HER2 status was verified by biopsies, and the metastases were detected by ^{18}F-FDG PET/CT 5 days before ^{111}In-ABY-025 imaging.[22]

^{111}In-ABY-025 produced high-contrast SPECT images within 4 to 24 hours. No anti-ABY-025 antibodies were observed ex vivo, indicating a non-immunogenic radiotracer, which is optimal for clinical translation. Background tissue uptake was highest in the kidneys, then the liver and spleen. ^{111}In-ABY-025 shows promise as a noninvasive tool for detecting HER2 in metastatic breast cancer, even during the occurrence of HER2-targeted antibody treatment.

Sandström and colleagues[21] produced a ^{68}Ga-labeled ABY-025 for diagnosis of HER2-positive breast cancer tumors with PET. The aim of the preliminary study with ^{68}Ga-ABY-025 was to measure the biodistribution and estimate the radiation dosimetry of ^{68}Ga-ABY-025 for 2 different peptide mass doses in the same group of patients (**Fig. 11**). Eight patients with metastatic breast cancer were included in this study. Each patient received a 45-minute dynamic (abdominal) and 3 whole-body PET/CT scans at 1, 2, and 4 hours after injection of a low peptide dose and a high peptide dose. The highest background uptake was observed in the kidneys and liver at all imaging time points.

In a phase I/II study, ^{68}Ga-ABY-025 to study effect of peptide mass and the effects on quantified uptake in tumors to pathologic analysis.[24] Sixteen women with metastatic breast cancer (confirmed by ^{18}F-FDG PET/CT) and receiving treatment were included. PET imaging was performed at 1, 2, and 4 hours after injection of 212 ± 46 MBq ^{68}Ga-ABY-025 (**Fig. 12** for example).

In the cohort of patients (10 total, 6 with HER2-positive, and 4 with HER2-negative primary tumors), ^{68}Ga-ABY-025 PET/CT with 2 different doses of injected peptide was performed. The optimal time

◀——————————————

^{68}Ga-HER2-nanobody. (*B*) Patient 12, injected with 0.1 mg. (*C*) Patient 17, injected with 1.0 mg. (*From* Keyaerts M, Xavier C, Heemskerk J, et al. Phase I study of 68Ga-HER2-nanobody for PET/CT assessment of HER2 expression in breast carcinoma. J Nuc Med 2016;57(1):30; with permission.)

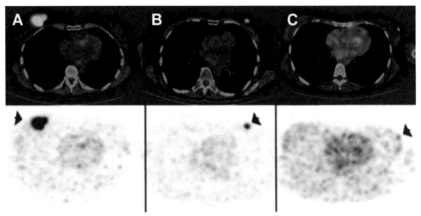

Fig. 15. Uptake of gallium-68 (^{68}Ga)-human epidermal growth factor receptor 2-nanobody in primary breast carcinoma lesions (*arrows*) on PET/computed tomography (CT) images (*top*) and PET images (*bottom*). (*A*) Patient 14 showed highest tracer uptake (mean standardized uptake value, 11.8). (*B*) Patient 15 showed moderate tracer uptake, which was easily discernable from background (mean standardized uptake value, 4.9). (*C*) Patient 6 showed no uptake (mean standardized uptake value, 0.9), with CT showing marker clip at tumor region. (*From* Keyaerts M, Xavier C, Heemskerk J, et al. Phase I study of 68Ga-HER2-nanobody for PET/CT assessment of HER2 expression in breast carcinoma. J Nuc Med 2016;57(1):31; with permission.)

point for ^{68}Ga-ABY-025 PET was found to be 4 hours, and accurately quantifies whole-body HER2-receptor status in metastatic breast cancer, and showed a change in uptake among patients receiving targeted treatment in 3 of the 16 patients. Patients with widespread metastatic disease were used as an example of ^{18}F-FDG versus ^{68}Ga-ABY-025 PET (**Fig. 13**) to gauge the ability of the radiotracer to detect distant disease.

CLINICAL PET IMAGING WITH RADIOLABELED NANOBODIES
Gallium-68-Human Epidermal Growth Factor Receptor 2-Nanobody

Nanobodies directed against HER2 have also been developed as probes for molecular imaging. Nanobodies are produced from a heavy chain component of antibodies, are the smallest antigen-binding antibody fragments, and have ideal characteristics for PET imaging.[61]

Initial studies by Keyaerts and colleagues[62] assessed the safety, biodistribution, and dosimetry of a ^{68}Ga-HER2-Nanobody. In this study, 20 women with primary or metastatic breast carcinoma were injected with ^{68}Ga-HER2-Nanobody (average dose, 107 MBq) and dosimetry calculations were based from images obtained at 10, 60, and 90 minutes after tracer administration. Representative images of this study are shown in **Fig. 14**.

The tumor-targeting potential was assessed in primary and metastatic lesions. No adverse reactions to the tracer were recorded, and only 10% of injected dose remaining in the blood at 1 hour after injection. Background uptake was observed in the kidneys, liver, and intestines. Primary tumors were more variable in tracer accumulation (**Fig. 15**), whereas metastatic lesions showed specific, easily delineated tracer accumulation (**Fig. 16**).[62]

Overall, ^{68}Ga-HER2-Nanobody PET/CT is a well-tolerated procedure with a comparable radiation dose to other routinely used PET tracers. The biodistribution of this radiotracer is favorable, with the highest uptake in the kidneys, liver, and intestines but low background levels in all other organs, including where primary or metastatic disease is most often found. Tracer accumulation in HER2-positive metastases is high, can be easily distinguished from background tissues, and warrants further assessment in a phase II trial.

18F-Human Epidermal Growth Factor Receptor 2-Nanobody

Xavier and colleagues[63] have recently labeled the GMP-produced HER2-nanobody with ^{18}F with and shown success with tumor targeting preclinically. Specific uptake for HER2-positive xenografts (5.94 ± 1.17% IA/g, 1 hour after injection) was observed with high tumor-to-tissue ratios. [^{18}F]-anti-HER2-nanobody showed rapid clearance through the kidneys (4% IA/g at 3 hours post-injection). The probe was also able to image HER2-positive tumors when coadministered with trastuzumab, indicating the potential use of this tracer for patient selection and monitor patients undergoing therapy. With the success of this ^{18}F-labeled probe and the positive results from phase I/II ^{68}Ga-HER2-nanobody trials, this probe should enter the clinic with ease.

A B

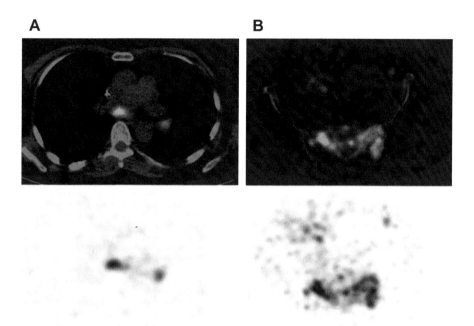

Fig. 16. Uptake of gallium-68 (^{68}Ga)-human epidermal growth factor receptor 2-nanobody in metastatic lesions on PET/computed tomography images (*top*) and PET images (*bottom*). (*A*) Patient 18, with invaded lymph nodes in mediastinum and left hilar region. (*B*) Patient 20, with bone metastasis in pelvis. (*From* Keyaerts M, Xavier C, Heemskerk J, et al. Phase I study of 68Ga-HER2-nanobody for PET/CT assessment of HER2 expression in breast carcinoma. J Nuc Med 2016;57(1):32; with permission.)

SUMMARY

HER2 receptor status is an important biomarker in patients with breast cancer, integral to treatment decisions and prognosis. HER2-targeted therapies have demonstrated clear survival advantages in patients with HER2-positive breast carcinoma. The possibility of heterogeneity of HER2 expression both within primary tumors and between primary and metastatic disease sites may limit the value of individual tumor biopsies and demonstrates a need for accurate, whole body assessment of HER2 status. Molecular imaging, most importantly PET, has been identified as a noninvasive tool to assess HER2-positive primary lesions and metastases. Radiolabeled antibodies, antibody fragments, and affibody molecules enable PET imaging to be a reliable and quantitative method for detecting HER2-positive cancer. HER2-targeted PET imaging has the potential to become a clinically valuable tool in the care of patients with breast cancer.

REFERENCES

1. Weigelt B, Peterse JL, van't Veer LJ. Breast cancer metastasis: markers and models. Nat Rev Cancer 2005;5(8):591–602.

2. Dunnwald LK, Rossing MA, Li CI. Hormone receptor status, tumor characteristics, and prognosis: a prospective cohort of breast cancer patients. Breast Cancer Res 2007;9(1):1–10.

3. van de Vijver M, Bilous M, Hanna W, et al. Chromogenic in situ hybridisation for the assessment of HER2 status in breast cancer: an international validation ring study. Breast Cancer Res 2007;9(5): R68–77.

4. Arteaga CL, Sliwkowski MX, Osborne CK, et al. Treatment of HER2-positive breast cancer: current status and future perspectives. Nat Rev Clin Oncol 2012;9(1):16–32.

5. Capala J, Bouchelouche K. Molecular imaging of HER2-positive breast cancer - a step toward an individualized "Image and Treat" strategy. Curr Opin Oncol 2010;22(6):559–66.

6. Elias SG, Adams A, Wisner DJ, et al. Imaging features of HER2 overexpression in breast cancer: a systematic review and meta-analysis. Cancer Epidemiol Biomarkers Prev 2014;23(8):1464–83.

7. O'Sullivan CC, Bradbury I, Campbell C, et al. Efficacy of adjuvant trastuzumab for patients with human epidermal growth factor receptor 2–positive early breast cancer and tumors ≤ 2 cm: a meta-analysis of the randomized trastuzumab trials. J Clin Oncol 2015;33(24):2600–8.

8. Paik S, Bryant J, Tan-Chiu E, et al. Real-world performance of HER2 testing—national surgical adjuvant

breast and bowel project experience. J Natl Cancer Inst 2002;94(11):852–4.

9. Becker S, Becker-Pergola G, Fehm T, et al. Her2 Expression on disseminated tumor cells from bone marrow of breast cancer patients. Anticancer Res 2005;25(3B):2171–5.

10. Perez EA, Suman VJ, Davidson NE, et al. HER2 testing by local, central, and reference laboratories in specimens from the north central cancer treatment group N9831 intergroup adjuvant trial. J Clin Oncol 2006;24(19):3032–8.

11. Paik S, Kim C, Wolmark N. HER2 status and benefit from adjuvant trastuzumab in breast cancer. N Engl J Med 2008;358(13):1409–11.

12. Ulaner GA, Hyman D, Ross D, et al. Detection of HER2-positive metastases in patients with HER2-negative primary breast cancer using the 89Zr-DFO-trastuzumab PET/CT. J Nuc Med 2016;57(10): 1523–8.

13. Tolmachev V. Imaging of HER-2 overexpression in tumors for guiding therapy. Curr Pharm Des 2008; 14(28):2999–3019.

14. Weissleder R. Molecular imaging in cancer. Science 2006;312(5777):1168–71.

15. Ulaner GA, Riedl CC, Dickler MN, et al. Molecular imaging of biomarkers in breast cancer. J Nuc Med 2016;57(Suppl 1):53S–9S.

16. Warram JM, de Boer E, Sorace AG, et al. Antibody based imaging strategies of cancer. Cancer Metastasis Rev 2014;33(0):809–22.

17. Lamberts LE, Williams SP, Terwisscha van Scheltinga AGT, et al. Antibody positron emission tomography imaging in anticancer drug development. J Clin Oncol 2015;33(13):1491–504.

18. Boerman OC, Oyen WJG. Immuno-PET of cancer: a revival of antibody imaging. J Nuc Med 2011;52(8): 1171–2.

19. van Dongen GA, Visser GW, Lub-de Hooge MN, et al. Immuno-PET: a navigator in monoclonal antibody development and applications. Oncologist 2007;12(12):1379–89.

20. Deri MA, Zeglis BM, Francesconi LC, et al. PET imaging with (89)Zr: from radiochemistry to the clinic. Nucl Med Biol 2013;40(1):3–14.

21. Sandström M, Lindskog K, Velikyan I, et al. Biodistribution and radiation dosimetry of the anti-HER2 affibody molecule 68Ga-ABY-025 in breast cancer patients. J Nuc Med 2016;57(6):867–71.

22. Sörensen J, Sandberg D, Sandström M, et al. First-in-human molecular imaging of HER2 expression in breast cancer metastases using the 111In-ABY-025 affibody molecule. J Nuc Med 2014;55(5):730–5.

23. Baum RP, Prasad V, Müller D, et al. Molecular imaging of HER2-expressing malignant tumors in breast cancer patients using synthetic 111In- or 68Ga-labeled affibody molecules. J Nuc Med 2010;51(6): 892–7.

24. Sörensen J, Velikyan I, Sandberg D, et al. Measuring HER2-receptor expression in metastatic breast cancer using [(68)Ga]ABY-025 affibody PET/CT. Theranostics 2016;6(2):262–71.

25. Kurihara H, Hamada A, Yoshida M, et al. 64Cu-DOTA-trastuzumab PET imaging and HER2 specificity of brain metastases in HER2-positive breast cancer patients. EJNMMI Res 2015;5(1):1–8.

26. Tamura K, Kurihara H, Yonemori K, et al. 64Cu-DOTA-trastuzumab PET imaging in patients with HER2-positive breast cancer. J Nucl Med 2013; 54(11):1869–75.

27. Mortimer JE, Bading JR, Colcher DM, et al. Functional imaging of human epidermal growth factor receptor 2–positive metastatic breast cancer using 64Cu-DOTA-trastuzumab PET. J Nucl Med 2014;55(1):23–9.

28. Slamon DJ, Leyland-Jones B, Shak S, et al. Use of chemotherapy plus a monoclonal antibody against HER2 for metastatic breast cancer that overexpresses HER2. N Engl J Med 2001; 344(11):783–92.

29. Romond EH, Perez EA, Bryant J, et al. Trastuzumab plus adjuvant chemotherapy for operable HER2-positive breast cancer. N Engl J Med 2005; 353(16):1673–84.

30. Breast cancer: trastuzumab therapy for small, HER2-positive breast tumours. Nat Rev Clin Oncol 2015;12(3):126.

31. Baselga J. Phase I and II clinical trials of trastuzumab. Ann Oncol 2001;12(Suppl 1):S49–55.

32. Buzdar AU, Ibrahim NK, Francis D, et al. Significantly higher pathologic complete remission rate after neoadjuvant therapy with trastuzumab, paclitaxel, and epirubicin chemotherapy: results of a randomized trial in human epidermal growth factor receptor 2–positive operable breast cancer. J Clin Oncol 2005;23(16):3676–85.

33. Dijkers ECF, Kosterink JGW, Rademaker AP, et al. Development and characterization of clinical-grade 89Zr-trastuzumab for HER2/neu immunoPET imaging. J Nuc Med 2009;50(6):974–81.

34. Gaykema SB, Schröder CP, Vitfell-Rasmussen J, et al. 89Zr-trastuzumab and 89Zr-bevacizumab PET to evaluate the effect of the HSP90 inhibitor NVP-AUY922 in metastatic breast cancer patients. Clin Cancer Res 2014;20(15):3945–54.

35. Dijkers EC, Oude Munnink TH, Kosterink JG, et al. Biodistribution of 89Zr-trastuzumab and PET imaging of HER2-positive lesions in patients with metastatic breast cancer. Clin Pharmacol Ther 2010;87(5):586–92.

36. Gaykema SB, Brouwers AH, Hovenga S, et al. Zirconium-89-trastuzumab positron emission tomography as a tool to solve a clinical dilemma in a patient with breast cancer: a case report. J Clin Oncol 2012; 30(6):e74–5.

37. Jhaveri K, Taldone T, Modi S, et al. Advances in the clinical development of heat shock protein 90 (Hsp90) inhibitors in cancers. Biochim Biophys Acta 2012;1823(3):742–55.

38. Friedland JC, Smith DL, Sang J, et al. Targeted inhibition of Hsp90 by ganetespib is effective across a broad spectrum of breast cancer subtypes. Invest New Drugs 2014;32(1):14–24.

39. Lavaud P, Andre F. Strategies to overcome trastuzumab resistance in HER2-overexpressing breast cancers: focus on new data from clinical trials. BMC Med 2014;12:132.

40. Gebhart G, Lamberts LE, Wimana Z, et al. Molecular imaging as a tool to investigate heterogeneity of advanced HER2-positive breast cancer and to predict patient outcome under trastuzumab emtansine (T-DM1): the ZEPHIR trial. Ann Oncol 2016;27(4):619–24.

41. University Medical Center Groningen, VU University Medical Center, University Medical Center Nijmegen. IMaging patients for cancer drug selecTion - metastatic breast cancer (IMPACT-MBC). In: ClinicalTrials.gov [Internet]. Groningen (The Netherlands): University Medical Center Groningen; 2016. NLM Identifier: NCT01957332. Available at: https://clinicaltrials.gov/ct2/show/NCT01957332. Accessed March 14, 2017.

42. Jules Bordet Institute. Pilot imaging study with 89Zr-trastuzumab in HER2-positive metastatic breast cancer patients (IJBMNZrT003). In: ClinicalTrials.gov [Internet]. Brussels (Belgium): Institut Jules Bordet; 2016. NLM Identifier: NCT01420146. Available at: https://clinicaltrials.gov/ct2/show/NCT01420146. Accessed March 14, 2017.

43. Jules Bordet Institute. HER2 Imaging Study to Identify HER2 positive metastatic breast cancer patient unlikely to benefit from T-DM1 (ZEPHIR). In: ClinicalTrials.gov [Internet]. Brussels (Belgium): Institut Jules Bordet; 2016. NLM Identifier: NCT01565200. Available at: https://clinicaltrials.gov/ct2/show/NCT01565200. Accessed March 14, 2017.

44. Memorial Sloan Kettering Cancer Center. United States Department of Defense, Genentech, Inc. Can HER2 targeted 89Zr-trastuzumab PET/CT identify unsuspected HER2 positive breast cancer metastases, which are amenable to HER2 targeted therapy?. In: ClinicalTrials.gov [Internet]. New York: Memorial Sloan Kettering Cancer Center (US); 2016. NLM Identifier: NCT02286843. Available at: https://clinicaltrials.gov/ct2/show/NCT02286843. Accessed March 14, 2017.

45. Washington University School of Medicine, National Cancer Institute (NCI). 89Zr Trastuzumab breast imaging with positron emission tomography. In: ClinicalTrials.gov [Internet]. St Louis (MO): Washington University School of Medicine (US); 2016. NLM Identifier: NCT02065609. Available at: https://clinicaltrials.gov/ct2/show/NCT02065609. Accessed March 14, 2017.

46. City of Hope Medical Center, National Cancer Institute (NCI). Copper (Cu) 64-DOTA-trastuzumab PET in predicting response to treatment with trastuzumab and pertuzumab before surgery in patients with HER2 positive breast cancer. In: ClinicalTrials.gov [Internet]. Duarte (CA): City of Hope Medical Center, (US); 2016. NLM Identifier: NCT02827877. Available at: https://clinicaltrials.gov/ct2/show/NCT02827877. Accessed March 14, 2017.

47. Perik PJ, Lub-De Hooge MN, Gietema JA, et al. Indium-111–labeled trastuzumab scintigraphy in patients with human epidermal growth factor receptor 2–positive metastatic breast cancer. J Clin Oncol 2006;24(15):2276–82.

48. Gaykema S, de Jong J, Perik P, et al. (111)In-trastuzumab scintigraphy in HER2-positive metastatic breast cancer patients remains feasible during trastuzumab treatment. Mol Imaging 2014;13:1–6.

49. Wong JYC, Raubitschek A, Yamauchi D, et al. A pretherapy biodistribution and dosimetry study of indium-111-radiolabeled trastuzumab in patients with human epidermal growth factor receptor 2-overexpressing breast cancer. Cancer Biother Radiopharm 2010;25(4):387–94.

50. Harbeck N, Beckmann MW, Rody A, et al. HER2 dimerization inhibitor pertuzumab – mode of action and clinical data in breast cancer. Breast Care (Basel) 2013;8(1):49–55.

51. Swain SM, Baselga J, Kim S-B, et al. Pertuzumab, trastuzumab, and docetaxel in HER2-positive metastatic breast cancer. N Engl J Med 2015;372(8):724–34.

52. Ontario Clinical Oncology Group (OCOG). Imaging with 111 indium (111In)-pertuzumab (PmAb) to predict response to trastuzumab (TmAb) in human epidermal growth factor-2 (HER2) positive metastatic breast cancer (MBC) or locally advanced breast cancer (LABC) (PETRA). In: ClinicalTrials.gov [Internet]. Hamilton (Canada): McMaster University, Ontario Clinical Oncology Group (Canada); 2016. NLM Identifier: NCT01805908. Available at: https://clinicaltrials.gov/ct2/show/NCT01805908. Accessed March 14, 2017.

53. Marquez BV, Ikotun OF, Zheleznyak A, et al. Evaluation of (89)Zr-pertuzumab in breast cancer xenografts. Mol Pharm 2014;11(11):3988–95.

54. Camel-IDS NV. Study to evaluate the safety, biodistribution, radiation dosimetry and tumor imaging potential of [131I]-SGMIB anti-HER2 VHH1 in healthy volunteers and breast cancer patients (CAM-VHH1). In: ClinicalTrials.gov [Internet]. Brussels (Belgium): Camel-IDS NV; 2016. NLM Identifier: NCT02683083. Available at: https://clinicaltrials.gov/ct2/show/NCT02683083. Accessed March 14, 2017.

55. Merrimack Pharmaceuticals. MM-302 plus trastuzumab vs. chemotherapy of physician's choice plus

trastuzumab in HER2-positive locally advanced/metastatic breast cancer patients (HERMIONE). In: ClinicalTrials.gov [Internet]. Cambridge (MA): Merrimack Pharmaceuticals (US); 2016. NLM Identifier: NCT02213744. Available at: https://clinicaltrials.gov/ct2/show/NCT02213744. Accessed March 14, 2017.

56. Merrimack Pharmaceuticals. Safety and pharmacokinetic study of MM-302 in patients with advanced breast cancer. In: ClinicalTrials.gov [Internet]. Cambridge (MA): Merrimack Pharmaceuticals (US); 2016. NLM Identifier: NCT01304797. Available at: https://clinicaltrials.gov/ct2/show/NCT01304797. Accessed March 14, 2017.

57. University of California, San Francisco. 64-Cu labeled brain PET/MRI for MM-302 in advanced HER2+ cancers with brain mets. In: ClinicalTrials.gov [Internet]. San Francisco (CA): University of California, San Francisco (US); 2016. NLM Identifier: NCT02735798. Available at: https://clinicaltrials.gov/ct2/show/NCT02735798. Accessed March 14, 2017.

58. Beylergil V, Morris PG, Smith-Jones PM, et al. Pilot study of (68)Ga-DOTA-F(ab')(2)-trastuzumab in patients with breast cancer. Nucl Med Commun 2013; 34(12):1157–65.

59. Weber WA. Chaperoning drug development with PET. J Nuc Med 2006;47(5):735–7.

60. Feldwisch J, Tolmachev V. Engineering of affibody molecules for therapy and diagnostics. Methods Mol Biol 2012;899:103–26.

61. Chakravarty R, Goel S, Cai W. Nanobody: the "magic bullet" for molecular imaging? Theranostics 2014;4(4):386–98.

62. Keyaerts M, Xavier C, Heemskerk J, et al. Phase I study of 68Ga-HER2-Nanobody for PET/CT assessment of HER2 expression in breast carcinoma. J Nuc Med 2016;57(1):27–33.

63. Xavier C, Blykers A, Vaneycken I, et al. 18F-nanobody for PET imaging of HER2 overexpressing tumors. Nucl Med Biol 2016;43(4):247–52.

Imaging of Prostate-Specific Membrane Antigen Using [^{18}F]DCFPyL

Steven P. Rowe, MD, PhD[a],*, Michael A. Gorin, MD[b],
Martin G. Pomper, MD, PhD[a]

KEYWORDS

- DCFPyL • Prostate cancer • Radiopharmaceutical

KEY POINTS

- 2-(3-{1-carboxy-5-[(6-[^{18}F]fluoropyridine-3-carbonyl)-amino]-pentyl}-ureido)-pentanedioic acid, or [^{18}F]DCFPyL, is a radiofluorinated, small molecule inhibitor of prostate-specific membrane antigen (PSMA) that allows PET imaging of this important cancer target.
- In patients with metastatic prostate cancer (PCa), [^{18}F]DCFPyL PET/computed tomography has been shown to identify many more suspicious lesions than are visible with conventional imaging.
- Preliminary results also demonstrate that [^{18}F]DCFPyL has improved sensitivity compared with conventional imaging for lesion detection in patients with metastatic clear cell renal cell carcinoma (ccRCC).

INTRODUCTION

Although PCa is the most common noncutaneous malignancy in men,[1] the accurate imaging of this common disease has long proved difficult. The mainstays of conventional imaging for PCa include MR imaging, contrast-enhanced computed tomography (CT), and ^{99m}Tc-methylene diphosphonate bone scan (BS). Although considered the current state-of-the-art, these imaging techniques have failed to completely address several important clinical questions.[2,3] As a result, numerous molecular imaging agents have been developed in the attempt to improve the diagnostic yield of PCa imaging. These include radiotracers targeting fatty acid synthesis,[4,5] amino acid transport,[6] the androgen receptor,[7] and the bombesin receptor.[8] Among the most promising targets, however, is PSMA, a type II transmembrane glycoprotein that is nearly universally overexpressed by PCa epithelial cells and serves as a marker for disease aggressiveness.[9,10]

PSMA-targeted radiotracers radiolabeled with a variety of radionuclides have been reported, including ^{111}In,[11] ^{99m}Tc,[12] ^{123}I,[13] ^{89}Zr,[14,15] ^{68}Ga,[16–18] and ^{18}F.[19,20] The authors' group has primarily focused on PET radiotracers labeled with ^{18}F due to the intrinsic quantitative nature and high spatial resolution of PET images as well as the

Disclosure: Dr M.G. Pomper is a coinventor on a US patent covering [^{18}F]DCFPyL and as such is entitled to a portion of any licensing fees and royalties generated by this technology. This arrangement has been reviewed and approved by the Johns Hopkins University in accordance with its conflict of interest policies. Dr M.A. Gorin has received payment as a consultant for Progenics Pharmaceuticals, Inc, the licensee of [^{18}F]DCFPyL. All authors have received research funding and salary support from Progenics Pharmaceuticals.
[a] The Russell H. Morgan Department of Radiology and Radiological Science, Johns Hopkins University School of Medicine, 600 North Wolfe Street, Baltimore, MD 21287, USA; [b] Department of Urology, The James Buchanan Brady Urological Institute, Johns Hopkins University School of Medicine, 600 North Wolfe Street, Baltimore, MD 21287, USA
* Corresponding author.
E-mail address: srowe8@jhmi.edu

near-ideal physical characteristics of ^{18}F relative to other PET radionuclides.[21–23] The culmination of the authors' group's efforts to date has been the clinical translation of the ^{18}F-labeled small molecule inhibitor of PSMA, [^{18}F]DCFPyL. This high-affinity compound has proved to provide very high tumor-to-background ratios and has allowed identifying putative sites of minimal disease across a range of clinical contexts. Furthermore, the authors have begun to explore the use of [^{18}F]DCFPyL in nonprostate cancers based on the known expression of PSMA in tumor-associated neovasculature.[24,25]

This article discusses the radiosynthetic approaches to [^{18}F]DCFPyL, preclinical developments using this molecule, and the initial experiences with early clinical studies in PCa and ccRCC.

RADIOSYNTHESIS OF [^{18}F]DCFPYL

[^{18}F]DCFPyL is based on a scaffold originally described by Kozikowski and colleagues[26] for targeting glutamate carboxypeptidase II within the brain. The first reported radiosynthesis of [^{18}F]DCFPyL in the literature is from Chen and colleagues.[27] They used a known radiofluorinated prosthetic group (6-[^{18}F]fluoronicotinic acid-2,3,5,6-tetrafluorophenyl ester, or [^{18}F]F-Py-TFP) to radiolabel a previously described asymmetric urea compound (**Fig. 1**A). With this methodology, decay-corrected radiochemical yields of [^{18}F]DCFPyL were in the range of 36% to 53% as based on the amount of [^{18}F]F$^-$ originally applied to the [^{18}F]F-Py-TFP synthesis, although relatively lower radiochemical yields have been reported in subsequent studies. Mean synthesis time was 128 minutes. Absolute yields with this synthetic approach were 285 MBq to 385 MBq (7.7–10.4 mCi) and specific activities were in the range of 12.6 GBq/μmol to 17.8 GBq/μmol (340–480 Ci/mmol), although larger absolute yields were obtainable with this method, which was the first to be adopted for human trials.

Recently, improved radiosynthetic approaches to [^{18}F]DCFPyL have been reported (see **Fig. 1**B). Both of these approaches have focused on nucleophilic fluorination of a protected DCFPyL precursor with subsequent deprotection steps, carried out in automated synthesis modules. Bouvet and colleagues[28] described an automated synthesis of [^{18}F]DCFPyL that used activated [^{18}F]F$^-$ (obtained from a stepwise drying procedure) to displace a trimethylammonium leaving group (see **Fig. 1**B). An acid deprotection step yielded [^{18}F]DCFPyL with a total synthesis time of 55 minutes, a significant improvement over the originally published radiosynthetic route.[27]

Decay-corrected radiochemical yields with this methodology were 23% ± 5% with specific activities in the range of 80 GBq/μmol to 100 GBq/μmol (2160–2700 Ci/mmol).

Ravert and colleagues[29] have also described methodology for [^{18}F]DCFPyL radiosynthesis based on direct radiofluorination of the same trimethylammonium precursor (see **Fig. 1**B). This method was validated on 2 different automated synthesis platforms. A custom-made radiofluorination module allowed the radiosynthesis of an average of 20.8 GBq ± 3.4 GBq (562 mCi ± 91 mCi) with an average specific activity of 4.4 TBq/μmol ± 0.3 TBq/μmol (120 Ci/μmol ± 9.2 Ci/μmol), not corrected for decay. These values equated to a non–decay-corrected yield of 30.9% ± 3.0% and an average synthesis time of 66 minutes, a similar length of time to the Bouvet and colleagues[28] method. An ELIXYS (Sofie Biosciences, Culver City, California) automated radiosynthesis module produced an average of 13.8 GBq ± 7.4 GBq (372 mCi ± 199 mCi) with an average specific activity of 2.2 TBq/μmol ± 0.5 TBq/μmol (59.3 Ci/μmol ± 12.4 Ci/μmol). Non–decay-corrected yields with the ELIXYS module averaged 19.4% ± 7.8%, with a relatively longer average synthesis time of 87 minutes.

Taken together, these recent advances in the radiosynthesis of [^{18}F]DCFPyL confirm the potential to make large quantities of this radiotracer, an important consideration if [^{18}F]DCFPyL is to be widely disseminated and used at many centers.

PRECLINICAL STUDIES WITH [^{18}F]DCFPYL

The preclinical findings reported by Chen and colleagues[27] in the same article containing the original radiosynthesis demonstrated the significant potential of [^{18}F]DCFPyL. An in vitro PSMA inhibition assay generated a K_i of 1.1 nM ± 0.1 nM. The high binding affinity of [^{18}F]DCFPyL was further manifest in favorable biodistribution experiments with nonobese diabetic severe combined immunodeficient mice bearing PSMA expressing and nonexpressing flank tumor xenografts. The PSMA + PC3-PIP xenografts in these mice demonstrated very high uptake of radiotracer, with 46.7% ± 5.8% injected dose/gram at 30 minutes after injection, with minimal decrease in percentage injected dose/gram over time out to 4 hours postinjection. Relative to PSMA-PC3-flu xenografts, the tumor uptake in the PIP xenografts ranged from 40:1 to more than 1000:1 over the time course of the study. Small animal PET imaging of these mice showed very high uptake of radiotracer in the PSMA + PC3-PIP xenografts,

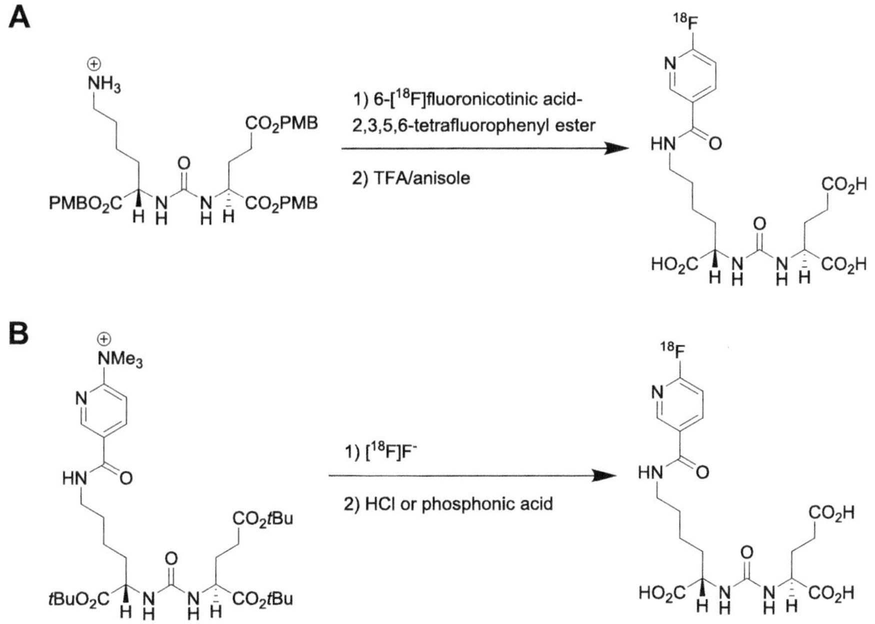

Fig. 1. Radiosynthetic approaches to [18F]DCFPyL. (*A*) The first published radiosynthesis[27] utilized the 6-[18F]fluoronicotinic acid-2,3,5,6-tetrafluorophenyl ester labeling group to install a radiofluorinated sidechain on an asymmetric urea, followed by an acid deprotection step. (*B*) More recently, 2 different groups[28,29] have reported improved radiochemical yields from [18F]F− displacement of a trimethylammonium leaving group urea precursor, again followed by an acid deprotection step. HCl, hydrochloric acid; PMB, *p*-methoxybenzyl; *t*Bu, *tert*-butyl; TFA, trifluoroacetic acid.

with no evidence of uptake outside of the xenografts by 3.5 hours postinjection.

Although the vast majority of effort with [18F]DCFPyL in recent years has focused on that clinical translation, the utility of the radiotracer as a preclinical imaging tool is still being explored. Airan and coworkers[30] recently described the use of MR imaging–guided focused ultrasound to open the blood-brain barrier in rats and allow access of highly hydrophilic agents into the central nervous system. [18F]DCFPyL was one of the molecules used for proof of principle for their study. Their results with dynamic small animal PET imaging showed the successful delivery of radiotracer to target in the brain.

CLINICAL APPLICATION OF [18F]DCFPYL IN PROSTATE CANCER

The initial experience with [18F]DCFPyL in humans consisted of a 9-patient, first-in-human prospective trial that enrolled patients with known progressive metastatic PCa (**Fig. 2**).[20] The patient population was a mix of hormone-naïve and castration-resistant men. Based on animal dosimetry estimates derived from the work of Chen and colleagues,[27] patients were administered a maximum of 333 MBq (9 mCi) of radiotracer and

were subsequently imaged at multiple time points to establish the biodistribution data needed to arrive at human dosimetry. The human dosimetry demonstrated that the kidneys received the highest estimated mean radiation dose (0.0945 mGy/MBq), with the urinary bladder wall (0.0864 mGy/MBq), submandibular glands (0.0387 mGy/MBq), and liver (0.0380 mGy/MBq) also receiving significant doses. Additional sites of uptake with lower exposures included the lacrimal glands, parotid glands, spleen, and small bowel. Outside the normal biodistribution, presumed tumor uptake was noted to be very high with lean-body-mass corrected standardized uptake values higher than 100 in the most visibly evident lesions.

The first-in-human study further demonstrated the safety of the radiotracer. No severe adverse events occurred among the 9 patients. Three adverse events (all grade I by the National Cancer Institute Common Terminology Criteria for Adverse Events) were noted during the study, none of which were thought attributable to the administration of the radiotracer.

A secondary analysis of 8 of the patients in the first-in-human trial evaluated the ability of [18F]DCFPyL to detect lesions in comparison to conventional imaging with CT and BS.[31] A markedly increased number of lesions were visible on [18F]

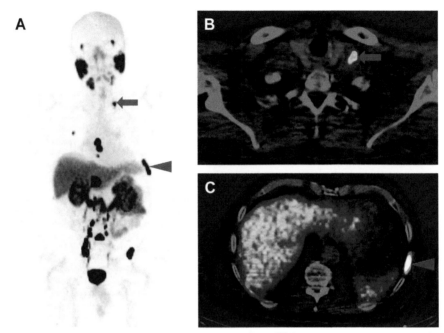

Fig. 2. (*A*) Whole-body maximum intensity projection image from [18F]DCFPyL PET in a patient with widespread metastatic PCa. Normal biodistribution includes lacrimal glands, salivary glands (this patient had a hypoplastic/ atrophic left submandibular gland), liver, spleen, kidneys, small bowel, ureters, and bladder. Block arrow demonstrates a left supraclavicular lymph node with intense radiotracer uptake that is shown in an axial PET/CT fusion image in (*B*). Arrowhead shows a rib lesion with intense radiotracer uptake that is also shown as an axial PET/CT image in (*C*).

DCFPyL PET/CT, with 138 definitive sites of abnormal radiotracer uptake and 1 additional site that was equivocal. In comparison, CT and BS together detected 30 definite sites suspicious for PCa involvement and an additional 15 that were equivocal. When taking into account intrapatient clustering effects through use of a general estimating equation regression model, it was estimated that a proportion of 0.72 of the lesions that would be negative or equivocal with conventional imaging would be definitively positive with [18F]DCFPyL PET/CT, whereas only an estimated proportion of 0.03 of the lesions that would be negative or equivocal with [18F]DCFPyL PET/CT would be definitively positive on conventional imaging. These findings were further supported in a case report comparing [18F]DCFPyL PET/CT to Na18 F PET/CT and BS in a patient with extensive bone metastatic PCa in which PSMA-targeted imaging detected several putative sites of disease that were occult with the bone-specific radiotracers.[32]

The work of Dietlein and colleagues[33] with [18F] DCFPyL has also showcased the sensitivity of this radiotracer for the detection of lesions in patients with PCa; 14 patients with elevated prostate-specific antigen levels after initial therapy for PCa were imaged with both [18F]DCFPyL

PET/CT and PET/CT with a 68Ga-labeled small molecule inhibitor of PSMA, [68Ga]Ga-PSMA-HBED-CC.[34] Although both radiotracers were able to identify sites of radiotracer uptake that were suspicious for disease in 10/14 (71%) patients, additional sites of putative disease were identified by [18F]DCFPyL in 3 patients. The improved lesion detection efficiency of [18F] DCFPyL relative to the 68Ga-labeled agent may reflect the intrinsic advantages of 18F as a PET radionuclide that were alluded to earlier.[21–23]

CLINICAL APPLICATION OF [18F]DCFPYL IN RENAL CELL CARCINOMA

Beyond its applications in PCa, the expression of PSMA in non-PCa tumor neovasculature that has long been established in the pathology literature[24,25] suggested that [18F]DCFPyL would be able to image effectively other tumor types. The authors' group has primarily focused on ccRCC due to its high degree of neovascularization (**Fig. 3**). In a pilot study of 5 patients with known metastatic ccRCC, [18F]DCFPyL PET/CT demonstrated a higher efficiency of lesion detection than conventional imaging, with 28 sites of discrete abnormal radiotracer uptake versus 18 sites suspicious for metastatic ccRCC identified

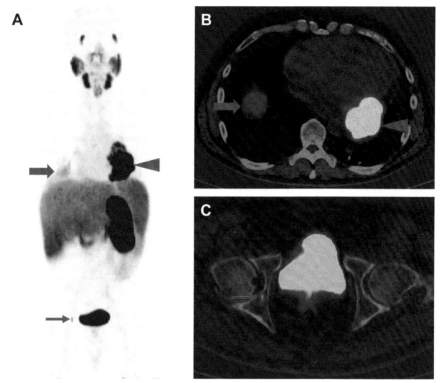

Fig. 3. (A) Whole-body maximum intensity projection image from [^{18}F]DCFPyL PET in a patient with metastatic ccRCC. Block arrow and arrowhead demonstrate bilateral lung masses; the right lung base lesion (*block arrow*) had previously been treated with external beam radiotherapy, likely explaining its lower uptake relative to the untreated left-sided lesion (*arrowhead*). (B) Axial [^{18}F]DCFPyL PET/CT fused image through the level of the lung lesions. The thin arrow in (A) points to a subtle bone lesion that was occult on CT but is well demonstrated on axial PET/CT (C).

on conventional imaging.[35] Eleven [^{18}F]DCFPyL-avid lesions were occult on conventional imaging, whereas contrast-enhanced CT had identified a liver lesion in 1 patient that was not appreciable on [^{18}F]DCFPyL PET/CT. Assuming that all sites of radiotracer uptake were truly positive, the sensitivity of [^{18}F]DCFPyL PET/CT in this study was 94.7%, compared with 78.9% for conventional imaging.

These findings in ccRCC were further supported by 2 subsequent case reports. The first involved a comparison of 1 patient who had PET/CT imaging with both the standard oncology radiotracer 2-deoxy-2-[^{18}F]fluoro-D-glucose ([^{18}F]FDG) and [^{18}F]DCFPyL.[36] [^{18}F]DCFPyL identified more lesions than [^{18}F]FDG, and in those lesions identified by both agents, uptake with [^{18}F]DCFPyL was demonstrably higher than uptake with [^{18}F]FDG. The second case report correlated areas of radiotracer uptake to pathology findings in a patient with widespread metastatic ccRCC who underwent a rapid autopsy approximately 1 month after imaging with [^{18}F]DCFPyL PET/CT.[37] In this patient, PSMA-targeted imaging identified 66

putative sites of disease. Of these, 12 were occult on conventional imaging with contrast-enhanced CT. Eight of these lesions were sampled during the autopsy and 7 (87.5%) were found definitively positive for metastatic ccRCC. A single bone lesion in a rib could not be confirmed pathologically. Together, these data support a role for [^{18}F]DCFPyL PET/CT imaging in ccRCC that is being further investigated in a larger study (Clinical-Trials.gov identifier NCT02687139). Outside of high sensitivity and specificity, the role of a neovascular imaging agent, such as [^{18}F]DCFPyL, in predicting response to neovascular-targeted agents, such as tyrosine kinase inhibitors, remains to be elucidated.

PITFALLS OF [^{18}F]DCFPYL IMAGING

As with any imaging test, [^{18}F]DCFPyL PET/CT does have limitations and pitfalls. The authors' group recently performed a correlation between imaging findings with [^{18}F]DCFPyL PET/CT, immunohistochemical analysis, and genomic findings in a patient with neuroendocrine dedifferentiated

PCa.[38] In a patient with long-standing metastatic PCa, pathologic samples were obtained from a peritoneal implant that had demonstrated low-level [18F]DCFPyL uptake and a liver lesion that had no discernable uptake. On immunohisto-chemical analysis, the peritoneal lesion stained moderately for PSMA whereas the liver lesion lacked any detectable PSMA. Genome-level analysis found that the peritoneal tumor was negative for synaptophysin and positive for NKX3.1 and CD56, indicating some measure of neuroendo-crine dedifferentiation but with some retained characteristics of typical prostate adenocarci-noma. In contrast, the liver lesion was frankly neuroendocrine in nature with the nonsense RB1 mutation E413X and the missense TP53 mutation I195 T. In total, these findings confirmed earlier findings that suggested PSMA-targeted imaging would be unable to reliably identify neuroendo-crine PCa,[39] indicating that patients with such tumors would be better imaged by other modalities.

An additional pitfall that has now been described in multiple case reports is the uptake of PSMA agents in Paget disease of bone.[40–43] The authors have also seen this phenomenon with [18F]DCFPyL PET/CT in a patient with bio-chemically recurrent PCa undergoing restaging examination.[44] Although pathologic proof of Paget disease was not sought in the case re-ported by the authors' group, the imaging fea-tures on CT, BS, and MR imaging were considered incontrovertible.

SUMMARY

Among the many new molecular imaging agents for PCa, [18F]DCFPyL demonstrates particular promise given its high affinity for the nearly univer-sally expressed target molecule PSMA, its labeling with the 18F radionuclide, and recent advances in its radiosynthesis that suggest large-scale pro-duction is feasible. [18F]DCFPyL PET/CT has also demonstrated excellent lesion detection sensitivity and specificity in patients with ccRCC. Although early clinical results are promising, additional larger prospective trials are needed to prove the utility of this new agent.

ACKNOWLEDGMENTS

The authors gratefully acknowledge support from NIH CA124675, CA184228, and CA183031 and the Prostate Cancer Foundation Young Inves-tigator Award, which have all contributed to the authors' ability to study [18F]DCFPyL and PSMA-targeted imaging.

REFERENCES

1. Siegel RL, Miller KD, Jemal A. Cancer statistics, 2016. CA Cancer J Clin 2016;66(1):7–30.
2. Maurer T, Eiber M, Schwaiger M, et al. Current use of PSMA-PET in prostate cancer management. Nat Rev Urol 2016;13(4):226–35.
3. Rowe SP, Gorin MA, Allaf ME, et al. PET imaging of prostate-specific membrane antigen in prostate cancer: current state of the art and future chal-lenges. Prostate Cancer Prostatic Dis 2016;19(3):223–30.
4. Bauman G, Belhocine T, Kovacs M, et al. 18F-fluoro-choline for prostate cancer imaging: a systematic re-view of the literature. Prostate Cancer Prostatic Dis 2012;15(1):45–55.
5. Jadvar H. Prostate cancer: PET with 18F-FDG, 18F-or 11C-acetate, and 18F- or 11C-choline. J Nucl Med 2011;52(1):81–9.
6. Schuster DM, Votaw JR, Nieh PT, et al. Initial expe-rience with the radiotracer anti-1-amino-3-18F-fluorocyclobutane-1-carboxylic acid with PET/CT in prostate carcinoma. J Nucl Med 2007;48(1):56–63.
7. Beattie BJ, Smith-Jones PM, Jhanwar YS, et al. Phar-macokinetic assessment of the uptake of 16beta-18F-fluoro-5alpha-dihydrotestosterone (FDHT) in prostate tumors as measured by PET. J Nucl Med 2010;51(2):183–92.
8. Lears KA, Ferdani R, Liang K, et al. In vitro and in vivo evaluation of 64Cu-labeled SarAr-bombesin analogs in gastrin-releasing peptide receptor-expressing prostate cancer. J Nucl Med 2011;52(3):470–7.
9. Ross JS, Sheehan CE, Fisher HA, et al. Correlation of primary tumor prostate-specific membrane anti-gen expression with disease recurrence in prostate cancer. Clin Cancer Res 2003;9(17):6357–62.
10. Perner S, Hofer MD, Kim R, et al. Prostate-specific membrane antigen expression as a predictor of prostate cancer progression. Hum Pathol 2007;38(5):696–701.
11. Manyak MJ. Indium-111 capromab pendetide in the management of recurrent prostate cancer. Expert Rev Anticancer Ther 2008;8(2):175–81.
12. Hillier SM, Maresca KP, Lu G, et al. 99mTc-labeled small-molecule inhibitors of prostate-specific mem-brane antigen for molecular imaging of prostate cancer. J Nucl Med 2013;54(8):1369–76.
13. Barrett JA, Coleman RE, Goldsmith SJ, et al. First-in-man evaluation of 2 high-affinity PSMA-avid small molecules for imaging prostate cancer. J Nucl Med 2013;54(3):380–7.
14. Osborne JR, Green DA, Spratt DE, et al. A prospective pilot study of (89)Zr-J591/prostate specific membrane antigen positron emission to-mography in men with localized prostate cancer

undergoing radical prostatectomy. J Urol 2014; 191(5):1439–45.

15. Pandit-Taskar N, O'Donoghue JA, Durack JC, et al. A phase I/II study for analytic validation of 89Zr-J591 ImmunoPET as a molecular imaging agent for metastatic prostate cancer. Clin Cancer Res 2015; 21(23):5277–85.

16. Afshar-Oromieh A, Malcher A, Eder M, et al. PET imaging with a [68Ga]gallium-labelled PSMA ligand for the diagnosis of prostate cancer: biodistribution in humans and first evaluation of tumour lesions. Eur J Nucl Med Mol Imaging 2013;40(4):486–95.

17. Eiber M, Maurer T, Souvatzoglou M, et al. Evaluation of Hybrid (6)(8)Ga-PSMA Ligand PET/CT in 248 patients with biochemical recurrence after radical prostatectomy. J Nucl Med 2015;56(5):668–74.

18. Maurer T, Gschwend JE, Rauscher I, et al. Diagnostic efficacy of (68)Gallium-PSMA positron emission tomography compared to conventional imaging for lymph node staging of 130 consecutive patients with intermediate to high risk prostate cancer. J Urol 2016;195(5):1436–43.

19. Cho SY, Gage KL, Mease RC, et al. Biodistribution, tumor detection, and radiation dosimetry of 18F-DCFBC, a low-molecular-weight inhibitor of prostate-specific membrane antigen, in patients with metastatic prostate cancer. J Nucl Med 2012;53(12): 1883–91.

20. Szabo Z, Mena E, Rowe SP, et al. Initial evaluation of [(18)F]DCFPyL for prostate-specific membrane antigen (PSMA)-Targeted PET imaging of prostate cancer. Mol Imaging Biol 2015;17(4):565–74.

21. Sanchez-Crespo A. Comparison of Gallium-68 and Fluorine-18 imaging characteristics in positron emission tomography. Appl Radiat Isot 2013;76: 55–62.

22. Gorin MA, Pomper MG, Rowe SP. PSMA-targeted imaging of prostate cancer: the best is yet to come. BJU Int 2016;117(5):715–6.

23. Rowe SP, Drzezga A, Neumaier B, et al. Prostate-specific membrane antigen-targeted radiohalogenated PET and therapeutic agents for prostate cancer. J Nucl Med 2016;57(Suppl 3):90S–6S.

24. Chang SS, O'Keefe DS, Bacich DJ, et al. Prostate-specific membrane antigen is produced in tumor-associated neovasculature. Clin Cancer Res 1999; 5(10):2674–81.

25. Chang SS, Reuter VE, Heston WD, et al. Five different anti-prostate-specific membrane antigen (PSMA) antibodies confirm PSMA expression in tumor-associated neovasculature. Cancer Res 1999;59(13):3192–8.

26. Kozikowski AP, Nan F, Conti P, et al. Design of remarkably simple, yet potent urea-based inhibitors of glutamate carboxypeptidase II (NAALADase). J Med Chem 2001;44(3):298–301.

27. Chen Y, Pullambhatla M, Foss CA, et al. 2-(3-{1-Carboxy-5-[(6-[18F]fluoro-pyridine-3-carbonyl)-amino]-pentyl}-ureido)-pen tanedioic acid, [18F]DCFPyL, a PSMA-based PET imaging agent for prostate cancer. Clin Cancer Res 2011;17(24):7645–53.

28. Bouvet V, Wuest M, Jans HS, et al. Automated synthesis of [(18)F]DCFPyL via direct radiofluorination and validation in preclinical prostate cancer models. EJNMMI Res 2016;6(1):40.

29. Ravert HT, Holt DP, Chen Y, et al. An improved synthesis of the radiolabeled prostate-specific membrane antigen inhibitor, [18 F]DCFPyL. J Labelled Comp Radiopharm 2016;59(11):439–50.

30. Airan RD, Foss CA, Ellens NP, et al. Mr-guided delivery of hydrophilic molecular imaging agents across the blood-brain barrier through focused ultrasound. Mol Imaging Biol 2016;19(1):24–30.

31. Rowe SP, Macura KJ, Mena E, et al. PSMA-based [(18)F]DCFPyL PET/CT is Superior to conventional imaging for lesion detection in patients with metastatic prostate cancer. Mol Imaging Biol 2016; 18(3):411–9.

32. Rowe SP, Mana-Ay M, Javadi MS, et al. PSMA-based detection of prostate cancer bone lesions with (1)(8)F-DCFPyL PET/CT: a sensitive alternative to ((9)(9)m)Tc-MDP bone scan and Na(1)(8) F PET/CT? Clin Genitourin Cancer 2016;14(1): e115–8.

33. Dietlein M, Kobe C, Kuhnert G, et al. Comparison of [(18)F]DCFPyL and [(68)Ga]Ga-PSMA-HBED-CC for PSMA-PET imaging in patients with relapsed prostate cancer. Mol Imaging Biol 2015; 17(4):575–84.

34. Eder M, Schafer M, Bauder-Wust U, et al. 68Ga-complex lipophilicity and the targeting property of a urea-based PSMA inhibitor for PET imaging. Bioconjug Chem 2012;23(4):688–97.

35. Rowe SP, Gorin MA, Hammers HJ, et al. Imaging of metastatic clear cell renal cell carcinoma with PSMA-targeted (18)F-DCFPyL PET/CT. Ann Nucl Med 2015;29(10):877–82.

36. Rowe SP, Gorin MA, Hammers HJ, et al. Detection of 18F-FDG PET/CT occult lesions with 18F-DCFPyL PET/CT in a patient with metastatic renal cell carcinoma. Clin Nucl Med 2016;41(1):83–5.

37. Gorin MA, Rowe SP, Hooper JE, et al. PSMA-targeted 18F-DCFPyL PET/CT imaging of clear cell renal cell carcinoma: results from a rapid autopsy. Eur Urol 2017;71(1):145–6.

38. Tosoian JJ, Gorin MA, Rowe SP, et al. Correlation of PSMA-targeted 18F-DCFPyL PET/CT findings with immunohistochemical and genomic data in a patient with metastatic neuroendocrine prostate cancer. Clin Genitourin Cancer 2017;15(1): e65–8.

39. Chakraborty PS, Tripathi M, Agarwal KK, et al. Metastatic poorly differentiated prostatic carcinoma

with neuroendocrine differentiation: negative on 68Ga-PSMA PET/CT. Clin Nucl Med 2015;40(2): e163–6.

40. Artigas C, Alexiou J, Garcia C, et al. Paget bone disease demonstrated on (68)Ga-PSMA ligand PET/CT. Eur J Nucl Med Mol Imaging 2016;43(1): 195–6.

41. Blazak JK, Thomas P. Paget disease: a potential pitfall in PSMA PET for prostate cancer. Clin Nucl Med 2016;41(9):699–700.

42. Sasikumar A, Joy A, Nanabala R, et al. 68Ga-PSMA PET/CT false-positive tracer uptake in Paget dis-ease. Clin Nucl Med 2016;41(10):e454–5.

43. Bourgeois S, Gykiere P, Goethals L, et al. Aspecific uptake of 68GA-PSMA in Paget disease of the bone. Clin Nucl Med 2016;41(11):877–8.

44. Rowe SP, Deville C, Paller C, et al. Uptake of 18F-DCFPyL in Paget's disease of bone, an important potential pitfall in clinical interpretation of PSMA PET studies. Tomography 2015;1(2):81–4.

Theranostic Prospects of Gastrin-Releasing Peptide Receptor– Radioantagonists in Oncology

Theodosia Maina, PhD[a],*, Berthold A. Nock, PhD[a],
Harshad Kulkarni, MD[b], Aviral Singh, MD[b],
Richard P. Baum, Prof, MD, PhD[b]

KEYWORDS

- Gastrin-releasing peptide receptor targeting • Theranostics • Receptor antagonist
- ^{68}Ga-radiotracer • Prostate cancer • Breast cancer

KEY POINTS

- The overexpression of gastrin-releasing peptide receptors (GRPRs) in prostate and breast cancer provides opportunities for diagnosis and therapy with GRPR-directed radiopeptides.
- Radiolabeled analogues of amphibian bombesin have been developed for GRPR-targeted tumor diagnosis and therapy.
- GRPR-radioantagonists, although unable to internalize in cancer cells, show considerable advantages for tumor targeting in human over their agonist counterparts, such as higher biosafety and superior pharmacokinetics.
- Translational studies have highlighted the excellent tolerability and the high diagnostic value of GRPR-radioantagonists in patients with prostate and breast cancer.

INTRODUCTION

The advent of radiolabeled somatostatin analogues in the diagnosis and therapy for neuroendocrine tumors (NETs) has paved new avenues for a theranostic patient-tailored management of cancer.[1,2] The successful application of somatostatin analogues in the clinic has relied on the high-density expression of somatostatin subtype 2 receptors (sst_2) in NETs compared with healthy background tissues.[3,4] Likewise, other peptide receptors and receptor subtypes are overexpressed in other types of human tumors providing the molecular basis for diagnostic imaging and radionuclide therapies with radiolabeled peptide analogues.[5,6] Research in this area offers excellent opportunities to expand the clinical indications of theranostic radiopeptides beyond the boundaries of sst_2-positive NETs and to upgrade the current armory of clinical oncology with a wider range of new effective molecular tools.

Much attention has been directed to gastrin-releasing peptide receptors (GRPRs) because of their expression in high numbers in major human cancers, such as in prostate and breast cancer.[7–10] Specifically, high-density expression of GRPR has been shown in primary prostate cancer in contrast not only to surrounding healthy tissue but also to

Disclosure: Drs T. Maina and B.A. Nock participate in an AAA-contract on NeoBOMB1 and are coinventors in a patent owned by AAA. Drs H. Kulkarni, A. Singh, and R. Baum have nothing to disclose.
[a] Molecular Radiopharmacy, INRASTES, NCSR "Demokritos", Aghia Paraskevi, Athens 15310, Greece;
[b] Theranostics Center for Molecular Radiotherapy and Molecular Imaging, Zentralklinik Bad Berka, Bad Berka 99497, Germany
* Corresponding author.
E-mail address: maina_thea@hotmail.com

the hyperplastic prostate that remains devoid of GRPR expression.[11] Hence, early neoplastic events in the prostate can be detected after administration of GRPR-directed peptide radiotracers with high specificity. In most cases, disease infiltrated to adjacent lymph nodes still retains a high GRPR-expression level, allowing for follow-up of metastatic spread. Yet, GRPR-expression seems to decline in advanced states of androgen-independent prostate cancer, especially when metastases involve the bone.[12–14] Likewise, in 60% to 75% cases of primary breast cancer, the GRPR is expressed at high densities with the expression levels fully retained in all lymph-node metastases originating from GRPR-positive primaries, allowing for follow-up of disease spread.[10,15,16] Other GRPR-positive cancers include lung cancer,[17–21] gastrinomas,[22] gastrointestinal stromal tumors,[23] as well as ovarian cancer whereby GRPR-expression is associated to tumor vasculature.[24,25]

In view of the above, much effort has been directed to the development of GRPR-seeking peptide radioligands.[26–28] Most of these analogues have been based on the amphibian tetradecapeptide bombesin (BBN, Pyr-Gln-Arg-Leu-Gly-Asn-Gln-Trp-Ala-Val-Gly-His-Leu-Met-NH$_2$) and its C-terminal fragments still retaining the ability to recognize and interact with the GRPR. Alternatively, C-terminal fragments of the 27mer gastrin-releasing peptide (GRP) (Val-Pro-Leu-Pro-Ala-Gly-Gly-Gly-Thr-Val-Leu-Thr-Lys-Met-Tyr-Pro-Arg-Gly-Asn-His-Trp-Ala-Val-Gly-His-Leu-Met-NH$_2$) native in mammals, for example, GRP(18–27) or neuromedin C, have likewise served as motifs for the development of GRPR-specific peptide radioligands.[29–31] Frog BBN binds both the GRPR and the neuromedin B receptor with equal affinity, whereas the human sequences are GRPR preferring.[7] Usually, peptide analogues of the aforementioned motifs have been further modified by covalent coupling of a bifunctional chelating agent (BFCA) at the N-terminus, either directly or via a spacer, to allow for stable binding of clinically relevant radiometals. This approach has provided a plethora of GRPR-seeking radiopeptides proposed for diagnostic imaging with single-photon emission computed tomography (SPECT) (^{99m}Tc, ^{111}In)[14,32–34] or PET (^{68}Ga, ^{64}Cu)[35–38] and for radionuclide therapy with the use of beta (^{90}Y, ^{177}Lu)[39–41] or alpha emitters (^{213}Bi).[42]

It should be noted that native BBN- and GRP-based peptides will bind and activate the GRPR after injection in the living organism. Thus, by acting as receptor agonists they induce potent adverse effects, especially in the gastrointestinal system, which restrict their clinical applicability.[43–47] The severity of such effects would depend on several factors,

including receptor binding affinity and potency of each analogue, dose and route of administration, as well as metabolic stability and bioavailability. The recent advent of GRPR-directed radiopeptides with antagonistic profile at the GRPR has offered an elegant way to circumvent the major biosafety concerns raised by the application of GRPR-activating radioligands.[48] In the present brief review the authors discuss significant breakthroughs in the development of GRPR antagonists and their radiolabeled analogues. Furthermore, the authors present promising new data in favor of the clinical application of GRPR radioantagonists in nuclear oncology.

TOWARD GASTRIN-RELEASING PEPTIDE RECEPTOR ANTAGONISTS AND THEIR RADIOLABELED ANALOGUES FOR USE IN GASTRIN-RELEASING PEPTIDE RECEPTOR–EXPRESSING TUMOR IMAGING AND THERAPY

The BBN-like peptide agonists after systemic administration exert a wide spectrum of biological actions on binding and activation of the GRPR, such as the release of gastrointestinal peptide hormones, the stimulation of exocrine gland secretion, and the contraction of smooth musculature, all synergistically translating into potent adverse reactions in the gastrointestinal system.[43,45–47,49,50] Furthermore, they have been implicated in the pathogenesis of human cancers via autocrine routes on GRPR-positive tumor cells, such as small cell lung carcinomas, prostate, or breast cancer.[17,19,51–54] Based on these facts, the use of BBN-like peptide agonist motifs for the development of GRPR-directed radioligands for diagnosis and therapy in clinical oncology seems to be entangled with biosafety risks. In the case of radionuclide therapy, whereby higher amounts of peptide analogues are typically administered, these risks become considerable. Biosafety issues became clearly evident during the clinical validation of ^{177}Lu-AMBA (^{177}Lu-DOTA-Gly-4-aminobenzoyl-Gln-Trp-Ala-Val-Gly-His-Leu-Met-NH$_2$) as a candidate radiopharmaceutical in the GRPR-targeted treatment of human prostate cancer.[41,42,44] In view of the aforementioned information, research efforts have recently switched from the development of radiolabeled BBN-/GRP-based agonists to GRPR-radioantagonists.[48]

Further positive support in the pursuit of this new research direction has been offered by a parallel shift of paradigm in the field of somatostatin. Accumulating evidence has shown that radiolabeled somatostatin analogues with an antagonistic profile at the sst$_2$ outperform their agonist-based counterparts in animal models and most importantly also in patients.[55–58] Specifically, sst_2-radioantagonists have shown higher tumor uptake and faster background clearance, even from organs and body tissues with physiologic high sst_2-expression levels. The exact biological mechanisms at play synergistically contributing to the superior pharmacokinetic profile of sst_2-radioantagonists in vivo have not been fully understood yet. However, at the cellular level sst_2-antagonists tend to bind both active and inactive receptor populations on the surface of target cancer cells, thereby favoring a stronger tumor localization in vivo.[56] Selected sst_2-radioantagonists with improved biological features are currently undergoing clinical trials as candidate radiopharmaceuticals in the theranostic management of NETs and other sst_2-positive tumors.[57,58]

An additional asset in the development of GRPR-radioantagonists is the great number of GRPR-antagonists developed since many decades by peptide chemists with the aim to better unravel the pharmacology and the role of bombesin receptors in health and disease.[59] These analogues were designed and synthesized after site-directed structural modifications at several positions of the native BBN and GRP sequences, including amino acid substitutions, reduction of peptide bonds, or peptide-chain truncations. It soon became apparent that modifications directed toward the C-terminus of native peptide chains led to the most potent antagonists at the GRPR. Several of these analogues were subsequently evaluated for their antiproliferative activity in various GRPR-expressing cell lines, and selected compounds thereof were further tested as anticancer drugs in human GRPR-expressing tumors xenografted in mice.[60–66] These developments have provided a wealth of data on the design and assessment of potent GRPR antagonists that have played an instrumental role in the development of GRPR radioantagonists for theranostic application in patients with cancer. The authors further report on modifications toward GRPR antagonists fostering the evolution of GRPR radioantagonists with promising perspectives for clinical translation.

C-Terminal Alkylated-Amide [des-Met¹⁴] Bombesin Analogues

Previous experience from gastrin and cholecystokinin has shown that removal of the C-terminal amino acid and/or replacement of its side chain by an alkyl amide or an ester leads to potent receptor antagonists.[67,68] This approach has stimulated the development of many potent [des-Met¹⁴] BBN derivatives, terminating as primary or secondary amides, alkyl esters, or hydrazides.[59,69,70]

The metabolic stability of resulting analogues was soon suspected to affect potency assessments in cell lines and in animal models (see later discussion). For example, antitumoral effects of the receptor antagonist in human GRPR xenografts raised in mice were significantly stronger after injection in the tumor compared with systemic administration implying rapid metabolic degradation by proteases in vivo.[59,71] Accordingly, substitution of natural amino acids by their d-analogues, especially at the N-terminus and/or N-capping by acetyl or other groups enhanced analogue potencies, most probably by conveying higher resistance to amino proteases. Results from biological assays performed with a considerable number of C-terminal substituted [des-Met¹⁴]BBN analogues have revealed that the nature of substitution at the C-terminus was crucial not only for determining GRPR affinity but also to initiate a biological response. Thus, several [des-Met¹⁴]BBN analogues acted as agonists, partial agonists, or as potent antagonists, such as the ethyl ester and alkyl amide derivatives. In the case of [dPhe⁶] BBN(6–13)–alkylamides, the length of the alkyl chain was found to affect agonistic/antagonistic properties at the GRPR, with the ethylamide being a pure receptor antagonist, the propyl amide a partial agonist, and the butyl amide an agonist.[59]

Coupling of an acyclic tetraamine at the N-terminus of the potent GRPR-antagonist [dPhe⁶]BBN(6–13)-NHEt via a spacer-generated demobesin 1 suitable for labeling with the diagnostic SPECT radionuclide ⁹⁹ᵐTc.[72] The forming radioligand, [⁹⁹ᵐTc]demobesin 1, showed excellent and GRPR-specific localization in human prostate adenocarcinoma PC-3 xenografts in mice and rapid clearance from background, including the GRPR-rich mouse pancreas. This attractive behavior enhancing tumor-to-background ratios with time is consistent with receptor-antagonism as was later confirmed by functional assays in PC-3 and HEK293-GRPR cells.[48] In a similar approach, diethylenetriamine pentaacetic acid (DTPA) was coupled to [dTyr⁶] BBN(6–13)-NHEt or [Tyr⁵,dPhe⁶]BBN(5–13)-NHEt allowing for labeling with ¹¹¹In.[34] However, at that time the lack of internalization in GRPR-positive cells was considered a handicap of the two GRPR-antagonist ¹¹¹In radiotracers compared with other internalizing agonist-based radiopeptides in the study. Furthermore, data acquired from comparative biodistribution in pituitary tumor-bearing female rats were in favor of the receptor agonists.[73]

Aiming toward a theranostic use of GRPR-antagonists in clinical oncology, demobesin 1 was subsequently modified by replacement of the acyclic tetraamine unit by the universal chelator 1,4,7,10-tetraazacyclododecane-1,4,7,10-tetraacetic acid

(DOTA). Thus, the resulting peptide conjugate, SB3, was suitable for labeling with a broad palette of bivalent and trivalent radiometals.[74] Labeling with the PET radionuclide ^{68}Ga yielded [^{68}Ga]SB3 showing single-digit nanomolar affinity for the GRPR. The [^{67}Ga]SB3 surrogate displayed excellent in vivo distribution in PC-3 xenograft-bearing mice, with high uptake and good retention in the experimental tumors combined with a rapid washout from the background. Compared with [^{99m}Tc]demobesin 1, the PET tracer surpassed tumor uptake values in the same animal model and at all time points. Tumor retention in particular was clearly superior for [^{67}Ga]SB3 (27.1 ±0.9% ID/g) compared with [^{99m}Tc]demobesin 1 (5.4 ±0.7% ID/g) at 24 hours after injection. In a first group of 17 patients with disseminated prostate and breast cancer, administration of [^{68}Ga]SB3 elicited no adverse effects, as expected for a GRPR antagonist. First clinical data with [^{68}Ga]SB3 PET/computed tomography (CT) in these patients were encouraging, with lesions visualized in about 50% of the patients, despite their advanced disease and extended previous therapies. The number of positive [^{68}Ga]SB3 scans was found significantly higher in patients with early stage prostate and breast cancer. Therefore, the value of [^{68}Ga]SB3 PET/CT for staging, monitoring, and eventually patient stratification for radionuclide therapy with beta emitters is currently under investigation in patient groups with primary and therapy-naïve prostate cancer and is correlated with biopsy and GRPR-status results.[75]

To explore the theranostic prospects of SB3, labeling with ^{111}In (for SPECT) and with ^{177}Lu was successfully performed. Biological evaluation revealed unexpected differences between either [^{111}In]SB3 or [^{177}Lu]SB3 and [^{68}Ga]SB3, mostly related to in vivo metabolic stability.[76] Unlike [^{68}Ga]SB3 that remained practically stable in circulation, [^{111}In]SB3 and [^{177}Lu]SB3 were degraded faster in vivo and their uptake in PC-3 xenografts in mice was accordingly compromised. Previous studies with BBN-based radioligands revealed neutral endopeptidase (NEP) as a major player in their in vivo catabolism.[77,78] By coinjection of the potent NEP-inhibitor phosphoramidon (PA), in vivo stability was enhanced and tumor uptake notably improved in animal models.[79] Adopting this elegant approach, coinjection of [^{111}In]SB3 or [^{177}Lu]SB3 with PA led in both cases to radiopeptide stabilization in peripheral mouse blood. Notably, the tumor uptake of [^{111}In]SB3 or [^{177}Lu]SB3 during PA treatment reached similar levels to those achieved by metabolically robust [^{68}Ga]SB3 in the same animal model, highlighting the importance of in vivo metabolic stability for successful tumor targeting.[76]

In another approach, the DTPA chelator was coupled via a spacer at the N-terminus of [dPhe^6]BBN(6–13)-NHPr instead of [dPhe^6]BBN(6–13)-NHEt to allow for labeling with ^{111}In.[80] The propylamide was previously reported for a higher affinity to GRPR compared with the ethylamide, but it was also characterized as a partial receptor antagonist in functional assays.[69] Interestingly, the resulting radioligand ^{111}In-bompromide internalized poorly in PC-3 cells as expected for a GRPR radioantagonist. However, uptake in PC-3 xenografts in mice was significantly lower and rapidly declining compared with either [^{99m}Tc]demobesin 1[72] or any of [$^{67/68}$Ga/^{111}In/^{177}Lu]SB3,[74,76] although background clearance was very fast.[80] It would be interesting to investigate how the in vivo metabolic stability and bioavailability of ^{111}In-bompromide play a role in the suboptimal tumor uptake and retention. The agonistic-antagonistic character of this analogue warrants further investigation as well in different functional assays in addition to internalization experiments to assess its actual biosafety for human use.

C-Terminal [Sta^{13},Met^{14}-NH$_2$]Bombesin Analogues

Potent GRPR antagonists could be obtained by replacement of the C-terminal Leu^{13}-Met^{14}-NH$_2$ dipeptide in the native BBN motif by Sta^{13}-Leu^{14}-NH$_2$ (statine, [3S, 4S]-4-amino-3-hydroxy-6-methylheptanoic acid).[59] This replacement in the BBN(6–14) fragment along with further substitution of Asn^6 by dPhe^6 yields the potent and GRPR-selective antagonist JMV594.[81,82] Modifications of JMV594 including the attachment of different BFCAs via a variety of spacers led to several analogues for radiolabeling with different radiometals for theranostic use in GRPR-positive human tumors.

Several examples of ^{68}Ga-/^{64}Cu-based radioligands[83–87] for PET, ^{111}In and ^{99m}Tc for SPECT,[88–90] as well as binding with the beta emitters ^{177}Lu[91,92] and ^{90}Y[93] for radionuclide therapy are briefly discussed later, and generated after coupling of DOTA via various chelators, such as PEG$_x$, βAla$_x$ and others.[88,89,94] Spacer length and type was found to affect GRPR-affinity and in vivo pharmacokinetics, with the introduction of positive-charged residues, such as the cationic spacer 4-amino-1-carboxymethyl-piperidine linker in RM2, shown to improve tumor uptake of resulting radioligands.[95] The impact of positive charge residues beyond the N-terminal of BBN(6–14)-like peptides has been studied previously with regards to the presence of basic Arg^{17} and Lys^{13} in the native human GRP and Arg^3 in amphibian BBN sequences.[31] This observation is in agreement with the higher GRPR-affinity and tumor uptake reported for N-terminal mono-cationic ^{99m}Tc-tetraamine chelate-carrying radiotracers, derived either from native BBN-/GRP-sequences[14,29,30,32,96] or from JMV594[90] and different types of GRPR antagonists.[72]

Owing to excellent pharmacokinetics in preclinical animal models, [^{68}Ga]RM2 was first evaluated in a group of 11 patients with prostate cancer with early stage disease applying PET/CT.[97] The tracer was very well tolerated by all patients and accurately visualized prostate-confined cancer, with its feasibility to depict metastatic lesions requiring further evaluation. In a subsequent study, [^{68}Ga]RM2 was studied in a group of 7 patients with recurrent prostate cancer in comparison with the prostate-specific membrane antigen (PSMA)-inhibitor ^{68}Ga–PSMA-11 (Glu-NH-CO-NH-Lys-[Ahx]-[^{68}Ga(HBED-CC)]).[98] This PET tracer can detect prostate cancer relapses and metastases by binding to a different pathologic lesion-associated target, namely, the extracellular domain of PSMA.[99] As expected for a non–GRPR-activating antagonist, [^{68}Ga]RM2 was well tolerated by all patients in accordance with previous findings. Unexpectedly, in this small patient cohort [^{68}Ga]RM2 was able to detect most metastatic lesions and in 2 cases also lesions missed by ^{68}Ga-PSMA-11. This first comparative study has highlighted the need for a further thorough investigation of GRPR and PSMA expression patterns in metastatic prostate cancer with the aim to more effectively exploit the combined theranostic potential of radioligands that interact with either or both of these molecular targets (see later discussion).[98]

The respective therapeutic [^{177}Lu]RM2 agent was next tested in a PC-3 xenograft mouse model alone or in combination with rapamycin,[91] a potent and specific inhibitor of protein kinase mammalian target of rapamycin.[100] In both cases [^{177}Lu]RM2 was found to be efficacious in inhibiting in vivo tumor growth, although uptake in the tumor was inferior compared with [^{68}Ga]RM2. In a recent study, [^{68}Ga]RM2 was shown to degrade by 50% within 15 minutes after injection in peripheral mouse blood.[101] Coadministration of PA led to full stabilization of the radiotracer in mouse circulation, directly implicating NEP in its in vivo catabolism and corroborating previous results.[79] The impact of the PA-induced stabilization on PC-3 tumor uptake was not investigated thoroughly in this case. In human [^{68}Ga]RM2 showed considerable degradation in circulation as well, with the intact radiotracer declining from $92 \pm 9\%$ at 1 minute to $19 \pm 2\%$ at 65 minutes after injection.[102] Based on these and previous findings,[76,79] it is reasonable to assume that the in vivo

performance of [^{68}Ga]RM2 and [^{177}Lu]RM2 is partly compromised by the action of NEP. This assumption was further supported by results from a recent study on the theranostic potential of [^{68}Ga/^{177}Lu]JMV4168 ([^{68}Ga/^{177}Lu]DOTA-(βAla)$_2$-JMV594) in preclinical prostate cancer animal models.[92] The coinjection of PA improved not only the intensity of [^{68}Ga]JMV4168 PET-signal on the experimental tumor but most importantly the therapeutic efficacy of [^{177}Lu]JMV4168 in mice, compared with non–PA-treated controls. Likewise, [^{111}In]JMV4168[89] in combination with PA was shown to more efficiently visualize 2 types of GRPR-expressing breast cancer xenografts in mice with SPECT/CT versus non–PA-treated animals.[16] These results further underscore the need for in vivo metabolically robust radioligands for maximizing delivery and optimizing uptake on tumor targets and, thereby, either image quality or therapeutic outcome.

Another interesting development toward therapeutic GRPR-radioantagonists involves the beta emitter ^{90}Y, previously used with success in radioimmunotherapy[103] as well as in the treatment of NETs with the aid of somatostatin analogues, such as DOTA-TATE and DOTA-TOC.[104,105] After coupling of DOTA via a polyethylene glycol 4 (PEG$_4$) spacer to the N-terminus of JMV594, and labeling with ^{90}Y, the biodistribution and dosimetry of the resulting ^{90}Y-AR radioligand was studied in mice bearing PC-3 xenografts.[106] In view of the absence of suitable γ emissions during ^{90}Y decay and the low abundance of positron emissions dosimetry becomes challenging. In an innovative strategy Cerenkov luminescence imaging was successfully used to determine radiation doses in mice. However, doses on the implanted tumor turned out to be inadequate for radionuclide therapy as a result of extensive radiolabel washout at time points beyond 4 hours after injection. To circumvent this handicap ^{90}Y-AR was applied in combination with vascular-targeted photodynamic therapy (VTP).[93] The latter is a local ablation approach recently approved for use in early-stage prostate cancer, generating reactive oxygen/nitrogen species within tumor blood vessels and leading to their instantaneous destruction followed by rapid tumor necrosis. Interestingly, VTP provided a successful means to trap ^{90}Y-DOTA-AR in the tumor microenvironment, thereby enhancing retention and therapeutic efficacy versus ^{90}Y-DOTA-AR monotherapy control mice.

In parallel, research has been directed as well in the development of ^{64}Cu-based JMV594 analogues for theranostic application in GRPR-expressing human cancer taking into account an appealing set of ^{64}Cu decay characteristics. Thus, in addition to its beta emission useful for therapy, ^{64}Cu simultaneously decays via positron emission suitable for PET imaging and dosimetry studies. Another attractive feature of ^{64}Cu is the intermediate half-life of 12.7 hours offering the possibility to investigate longer processes in the body compared with shorter-lived PET radionuclides (^{18}F, ^{68}Ga). Besides DOTA several chelators suitable for stable binding of copper were coupled to the N-terminus of JMC594 via different spacers and were evaluated in preclinical models.[83,84] Among the new ^{64}Cu-labeled GRPR antagonists, ^{64}Cu-CB-TE2A-AR06 [(^{64}Cu-4,11-bis (carboxymethyl)-1,4,8,11-tetraazabicyclo(6.6.2) hexadecane)-PEG$_4$-dPhe-Gln-Trp-Ala-Val-Gly-His-Sta-Leu-NH$_2$] was studied by PET/CT in 4 patients with newly diagnosed prostate cancer.[107] The tracer was well tolerated by all patients. Three of 4 tumors were visualized with high contrast, and one small lesion with less than 5% tumor tissue on biopsy showed moderate contrast at 4 hours post injection, whereas radioactivity rapidly cleared from the background.

C-Terminal [des-Leu^{26},des-Met^{27}-Alkylamide] Gastrin-Releasing Peptide(20–27) Analogues

A series of very potent GRPR antagonists could be generated from human N-acetyl GRP(20–27) by truncation of the C-terminal Leu^{26}-Met^{27}-NH$_2$ dipeptide and modification of C-terminal carboxyl group of His^{25} with a variety of alkylamides.[59] These analogues were found resistant to enzymatic degradation in human serum and demonstrated strong binding affinity for the GRPR.[108] Of particular interest is N-acetyl-GRP(20–25)-NH-CH[CH$_2$-CH(CH$_3$)$_2$]$_2$, displaying equipotent GRPR-binding affinity with native GRP and a strong antagonistic profile in 3 different functional assays. By adopting this C-terminal His^{25}-Leu^{26}-Met^{27}-NH$_2$ to His^{25}-NH-CH[CH$_2$-CH(CH$_3$)$_2$]$_2$ modification in the SB3 motif,[74] NeoBOMB1 was generated suitable for labeling with useful radiometals for theranostic management of GRPR-expressing human tumors.[109]

After binding of any of ^{111}In, ^{67}Ga (as ^{68}Ga surrogate), and ^{177}Lu, NeoBOMB1 preserved single-digit nanomolar affinity for the GRPR and showed high binding efficiency in GRPR-positive cells localizing mainly on the cell surface. All 3 [^{111}In/^{67}Ga/^{177}Lu] NeoBOMB1 radioligands independent of the radiometal used remained intact in peripheral mouse blood and showed very high uptake and good retention in experimental prostate and breast cancer tumors in mice.[109,110] Furthermore, by tuning the amount of peptide injected in mice, [^{177}Lu]Neo-BOMB1 uptake in physiologic GRPR-rich organs was significantly suppressed, improving dosimetry and highlighting the theranostic potential of Neo-BOMB1.[111] In a first-in-man study applying PET/ CT in a group of 4 patients in various stages of prostate cancer, [^{68}Ga]NeoBOMB1 strongly visualized primary prostate-confined disease but also multimetastatic foci during disease spread, such as liver micrometastases and bone lesions. The tracer displayed high lesion-to-background ratios and was well-tolerated by all patients in favor of potential clinical use of the respective [^{68}Ga/^{177}Lu] NeoBOMB1 theranostic pair in GRPR-positive cancer.[109–112]

THERANOSTIC PROSPECTS OF GASTRIN-RELEASING PEPTIDE RECEPTOR RADIOANTAGONISTS IN ONCOLOGY: CONCLUDING REMARKS

Theranostic approaches for GRPR-expressing human tumors, such as the frequently occurring prostate and breast cancer, are expected to enter the clinic in the near future as a result of the continuous emergence of state-of-the-art GRPR radioantagonists.[74,97,107,109] As shown in this brief survey, GRPR radioantagonists are associated to higher biosafety and potent targeting of tumor lesions combined with attractive pharmacokinetics in animal models and patients compared with agonists. These qualities, attractive for high-contrast imaging, have also raised hopes for safer and more efficacious radionuclide therapies, as soon as a few antagonist-related issues are addressed first: (1) Prolonged retention of a radioantagonist on GRPR-expressing cancer cells, in addition to a high GRPR affinity, is important for high therapeutic efficacy. Accordingly, the structural requirements and underlying mechanisms for sustained binding of GRPR radioantagonists on cancer cells need to be better understood and elegantly exploited.[91,93] (2) Equally significant is the in vivo metabolic stability of GRPR radioantagonists to ensure optimum radiolabel supply to tumor sites and thereby delivery of maximum radiotoxic loads on cancer cells.[76,92] (3) Eventually, the applicability of noninternalizing GRPR radioantagonists labeled with α-emitters for effective radionuclide therapy needs to be investigated in detail. Research on these topics is expected to intensify in the coming years.

Another factor potentially affecting the theranostic value of GRPR antagonists in clinical oncology concerns the GRPR overexpression in different human cancers, or in different stages of the same cancer. For example, the high-density GRPR expression in early stages of well-differentiated prostate carcinoma declines in more advanced androgen-independent stages of the disease with metastatic spread involving the bone. However, and despite the fact that excellent outcome in therapy-naïve patients has been already observed,[75,97] good tracer localization has been also demonstrated in several, but not all, prostate cancer skeletal lesions.[14,74,109] Thus, more clinical studies including more patients in metastasized bone disease are warranted to better understand the molecular basis for the high GRPR expression in some bone metastases versus the total lack of expression in others. Furthermore, imaging findings should be correlated with histology, androgen receptor status, and other factors.

In this respect, other molecular probes, like radiolabeled small-size PSMA inhibitors, may offer alternative or complementary theranostic tools in advanced less-differentiated prostate cancer.[113–115] In a recent study comparing PSMA- versus GRPR-directed ^{68}Ga-labeled probes applying PET/CT in 7 patients with prostate cancer, the aforementioned clear-cut concept seems not to apply in all lesion cases, demonstrating that the clinical implications of PSMA and GRPR expression as the disease propagates are not fully understood up to now. For this purpose, further comparative head-to-head clinical studies are warranted. A characteristic example in support of this requirement is the 69-year-old patient, with moderately differentiated Gleason 7 (4 + 3) prostate adenocarcinoma (initial tumor classification pT3a pN0(0/18) M0, L1 V0 Pn1, stage II,

UICC 2010) salvage radical prostatectomy and salvage conformal radiation therapy to prostate bed/pelvic lymph nodes and androgen deprivation therapy, presented to Zentralklinik Bad Berka with progressive multiple bone metastases and increasing PSA.

The patient initially underwent ^{68}Ga-PSMA PET/CT (Fig. 1A) to determine the PSMA expression level in the metastases for potential radionuclide therapy with ^{177}Lu-PSMA.[114,115] Unexpectedly, ^{68}Ga-PSMA PET/CT was negative with multiple bone metastases demonstrating no radiolabel uptake as a result of PSMA expression. In contrast, there was a significantly increased osteo-metabolism in multiple bone metastases visualized by ^{18}F-fluoride PET/CT (see Fig. 1B). On the other hand, ^{68}Ga-GRPR-antagonist PET/CT (see Fig. 1C) revealed GRPR expression in many of the osteoblastic metastases (matching with ^{18}F-fluoride PET/CT). Notably, a mismatch finding was also revealed (Fig. 2A1, A2) concerning a GRPR-positive bone marrow metastasis in the right humerus (see Fig. 2A1), negative on ^{18}F-fluoride PET/CT (see Fig. 2A2). However, almost all other metastases displayed predominantly osteoblastic changes with intense ^{18}F-fluoride uptake (Fig. 2B–E). The patient underwent therapy with

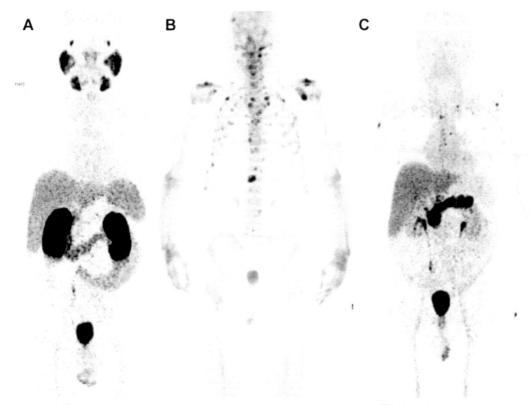

A   **B**   **C**

Fig. 1. (A) ^{68}Ga-PSMA PET/CT maximum intensity projection (MIP) image, (B) ^{18}F-fluoride PET/CT MIP image, and (C) ^{68}Ga-GRPR-antagonist PET/CT MIP image.

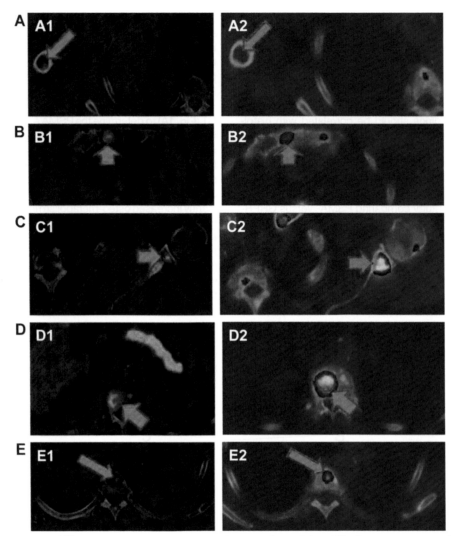

Fig. 2. (*A1–E1*) Fused ^{68}Ga-GRPR-antagonist PET/CT axial images; (*A2–E2*) fused ^{18}F-fluoride PET/CT axial images of metastases (indicated by the *blue arrows*) in right humerus (*A*), sternum (*B*), left scapula (*C*), and in the dorsal vertebrae (*D, E*).

the bone-seeking therapeutic radiopharmaceutical ^{177}Lu-BPAMD,[116] which exhibited an intense accumulation in bone metastases.

This case underlines once again the importance of combining different diagnostic tracers addressing distinctive functional characteristics of metastatic prostate cancer (and presumably also other GRPR-expressing cancers), namely, PSMA expression, osteo-metabolism, and GRPR expression, in order to select the most appropriate agent for therapy, based on the concept of theranostics.[113]

REFERENCES

1. de Jong M, Breeman WA, Kwekkeboom DJ, et al. Tumor imaging and therapy using radiolabeled somatostatin analogues. Acc Chem Res 2009;42:873–80.

2. van Essen M, Krenning EP, Kam BL, et al. Peptide-receptor radionuclide therapy for endocrine tumors. Nat Rev Endocrinol 2009;5:382–93.

3. Reubi JC, Krenning E, Lamberts SW, et al. Somatostatin receptors in malignant tissues. J Steroid Biochem Mol Biol 1990;37:1073–7.

4. Reubi JC, Waser B, Schaer JC, et al. Somatostatin receptor sst_1-sst_5 expression in normal and neoplastic human tissues using receptor autoradiography with subtype-selective ligands. Eur J Nucl Med 2001;28:836–46.

5. Reubi JC. Peptide receptors as molecular targets for cancer diagnosis and therapy. Endocr Rev 2003;24:389–427.

6. Reubi JC. Old and new peptide receptor targets in cancer: future directions. Recent Results Cancer Res 2013;194:567–76.

7. Kroog GS, Jensen RT, Battey JF. Mammalian bombesin receptors. Med Res Rev 1995;15:389–417.

8. Gonzalez N, Moody TW, Igarashi H, et al. Bombesin-related peptides and their receptors: recent advances in their role in physiology and disease states. Curr Opin Endocrinol Diabetes Obes 2008; 15:58–64.

9. Markwalder R, Reubi JC. Gastrin-releasing peptide receptors in the human prostate: relation to neoplastic transformation. Cancer Res 1999;59:1152–9.

10. Gugger M, Reubi JC. Gastrin-releasing peptide receptors in non-neoplastic and neoplastic human breast. Am J Pathol 1999;155:2067–76.

11. Körner M, Waser B, Rehmann R, et al. Early overexpression of GRP receptors in prostatic carcinogenesis. Prostate 2014;74:217–24.

12. Beer M, Montani M, Gerhardt J, et al. Profiling gastrin-releasing peptide receptor in prostate tissues: clinical implications and molecular correlates. Prostate 2012;72:318–25.

13. Schroeder RP, de Visser M, van Weerden WM, et al. Androgen-regulated gastrin-releasing peptide receptor expression in androgen-dependent human prostate tumor xenografts. Int J Cancer 2010;126:2826–34.

14. Mather SJ, Nock BA, Maina T, et al. GRP receptor imaging of prostate cancer using [^{99m}Tc]demobesin 4: a first-in-man study. Mol Imaging Biol 2014; 16:888–95.

15. Halmos G, Wittliff JL, Schally AV. Characterization of bombesin/gastrin-releasing peptide receptors in human breast cancer and their relationship to steroid receptor expression. Cancer Res 1995;55: 280–7.

16. Dalm SU, Martens JW, Sieuwerts AM, et al. In vitro and in vivo application of radiolabeled gastrin-releasing peptide receptor ligands in breast cancer. J Nucl Med 2015;56:752–7.

17. Cuttitta F, Carney DN, Mulshine J, et al. Bombesin-like peptides can function as autocrine growth factors in human small-cell lung cancer. Nature 1985; 316:823–6.

18. Moody TW, Carney DN, Cuttitta F, et al. High affinity receptors for bombesin/GRP-like peptides on human small cell lung cancer. Life Sci 1985;37: 105–13.

19. Cuttitta F, Carney DN, Mulshine J, et al. Autocrine growth factors in human small cell lung cancer. Cancer Surv 1985;4:707–27.

20. Moody TW, Zia F, Venugopal R, et al. GRP receptors are present in non small cell lung cancer cells. J Cell Biochem Suppl 1996;24:247–56.

21. Mattei J, Achcar RD, Cano CH, et al. Gastrin-releasing peptide receptor expression in lung cancer. Arch Pathol Lab Med 2014;138:98–104.

22. Reubi JC, Wenger S, Schmuckli-Maurer J, et al. Bombesin receptor subtypes in human cancers:

detection with the universal radioligand ^{125}I-[D-Tyr^6,beta-Ala^{11},Phe^{13},Nle^{14}]bombesin(6-14). Clin Cancer Res 2002;8:1139–46.

23. Reubi JC, Körner M, Waser B, et al. High expression of peptide receptors as a novel target in gastrointestinal stromal tumours. Eur J Nucl Med Mol Imaging 2004;31:803–10.

24. Sun B, Schally AV, Halmos G. The presence of receptors for bombesin/GRP and mRNA for three receptor subtypes in human ovarian epithelial cancers. Regul Pept 2000;90:77–84.

25. Fleischmann A, Waser B, Reubi JC. Overexpression of gastrin-releasing peptide receptors in tumor-associated blood vessels of human ovarian neoplasms. Cell Oncol 2007;29:421–33.

26. Moreno P, Ramos-Alvarez I, Moody TW, et al. Bombesin related peptides/receptors and their promising therapeutic roles in cancer imaging, targeting and treatment. Expert Opin Ther Targets 2016;20:1055–73.

27. Maina T, Nock B, Mather S. Targeting prostate cancer with radiolabelled bombesins. Cancer Imaging 2006;6:153–7.

28. Maina T, Nock BA. From bench to bed: new gastrin releasing peptide receptor-directed radioligands and their use in prostate cancer. PET Clinics 2017;12(2):205–17.

29. Nock BA, Cescato R, Ketani E, et al. [^{99m}Tc]demomedin C, a radioligand based on human gastrin releasing peptide(18-27): synthesis and preclinical evaluation in gastrin releasing peptide receptor-expressing models. J Med Chem 2012;55:8364–74.

30. Marsouvanidis PJ, Maina T, Sallegger W, et al. ^{99m}Tc radiotracers based on human GRP(18-27): synthesis and comparative evaluation. J Nucl Med 2013;54:1797–803.

31. Marsouvanidis PJ, Maina T, Sallegger W, et al. Tumor diagnosis with new ^{111}In-radioligands based on truncated human gastrin releasing peptide sequences: synthesis and preclinical comparison. J Med Chem 2013;56:8579–87.

32. Nock BA, Nikolopoulou A, Galanis A, et al. Potent bombesin-like peptides for GRP-receptor targeting of tumors with ^{99m}Tc: a preclinical study. J Med Chem 2005;48:100–10.

33. Breeman WA, De Jong M, Bernard BF, et al. Pre-clinical evaluation of [^{111}In-DTPA-Pro^1,Tyr^4]bombesin, a new radioligand for bombesin-receptor scintigraphy. Int J Cancer 1999;83:657–63.

34. Breeman WA, de Jong M, Erion JL, et al. Preclinical comparison of ^{111}In-labeled DTPA- or DOTA-bombesin analogs for receptor-targeted scintigraphy and radionuclide therapy. J Nucl Med 2002;43:1650–6.

35. Parry JJ, Kelly TS, Andrews R, et al. In vitro and in vivo evaluation of ^{64}Cu-labeled DOTA-linker-bombesin(7-14) analogues containing different

amino acid linker moieties. Bioconjug Chem 2007;
18:1110–7.

36. Biddlecombe GB, Rogers BE, de Visser M, et al. Molecular imaging of gastrin-releasing peptide receptor-positive tumors in mice using ^{64}Cu- and ^{86}Y-DOTA-(Pro^1,Tyr^4)-bombesin(1-14). Bioconjug Chem 2007;18:724–30.

37. Lane SR, Nanda P, Rold TL, et al. Optimization, biological evaluation and microPET imaging of copper-64-labeled bombesin agonists, [^{64}Cu-NO2A-(X)-BBN(7-14)NH$_2$], in a prostate tumor xenografted mouse model. Nucl Med Biol 2010;37: 751–61.

38. Prignon A, Nataf V, Provost C, et al. Ga-AMBA and F-FDG for preclinical PET imaging of breast cancer: effect of tamoxifen treatment on tracer uptake by tumor. Nucl Med Biol 2015;42:92–8.

39. Zhang H, Chen J, Waldherr C, et al. Synthesis and evaluation of bombesin derivatives on the basis of pan-bombesin peptides labeled with indium-111, lutetium-177, and yttrium-90 for targeting bombesin receptor-expressing tumors. Cancer Res 2004;64:6707–15.

40. Zhang H, Schuhmacher J, Waser B, et al. DOTA-PESIN, a DOTA-conjugated bombesin derivative designed for the imaging and targeted radionuclide treatment of bombesin receptor-positive tumours. Eur J Nucl Med Mol Imaging 2007;34: 1198–208.

41. Lantry LE, Cappelletti E, Maddalena ME, et al. ^{177}Lu-AMBA: synthesis and characterization of a selective ^{177}Lu-labeled GRP-R agonist for systemic radiotherapy of prostate cancer. J Nucl Med 2006; 47:1144–52.

42. Wild D, Frischknecht M, Zhang H, et al. Alpha-versus beta-particle radiopeptide therapy in a human prostate cancer model (^{213}Bi-DOTA-PESIN and ^{213}Bi-AMBA versus ^{177}Lu-DOTA-PESIN). Cancer Res 2011;71:1009–18.

43. Vigna SR, Mantyh CR, Giraud AS, et al. Localization of specific binding sites for bombesin in the canine gastrointestinal tract. Gastroenterology 1987;93:1287–95.

44. Bodei L, Ferrari M, Nunn A, et al. ^{177}Lu-AMBA bombesin analogue in hormone refractory prostate cancer patients: a phase I escalation study with single-cycle administrations. Eur J Nucl Med Mol Imaging 2007;34:S221.

45. Delle Fave G, Annibale B, de Magistris L, et al. Bombesin effects on human GI functions. Peptides 1985;6(Suppl 3):113–6.

46. Bruzzone R, Tamburrano G, Lala A, et al. Effect of bombesin on plasma insulin, pancreatic glucagon, and gut glucagon in man. J Clin Endocrinol Metab 1983;56:643–7.

47. Severi C, Jensen RT, Erspamer V, et al. Different receptors mediate the action of bombesin-related peptides on gastric smooth muscle cells. Am J Physiol 1991;260:G683–90.

48. Cescato R, Maina T, Nock B, et al. Bombesin receptor antagonists may be preferable to agonists for tumor targeting. J Nucl Med 2008;49:318–26.

49. Bitar KN, Zhu XX. Expression of bombesin-receptor subtypes and their differential regulation of colonic smooth muscle contraction. Gastroenterology 1993; 105:1672–80.

50. Rozengurt E, Sinnett-Smith J. Bombesin stimulation of fibroblast mitogenesis: specific receptors, signal transduction and early events. Philos Trans R Soc Lond B Biol Sci 1990;327:209–21.

51. Preston SR, Miller GV, Primrose JN. Bombesin-like peptides and cancer. Crit Rev Oncol Hematol 1996;23:225–38.

52. Chao C, Ives K, Hellmich HL, et al. Gastrin-releasing peptide receptor in breast cancer mediates cellular migration and interleukin-8 expression. J Surg Res 2009;156:26–31.

53. Aprikian AG, Han K, Guy L, et al. Neuroendocrine differentiation and the bombesin/gastrin-releasing peptide family of neuropeptides in the progression of human prostate cancer. Prostate Suppl 1998;8: 52–61.

54. Bologna M, Festuccia C, Muzi P, et al. Bombesin stimulates growth of human prostatic cancer cells in vitro. Cancer 1989;63:1714–20.

55. Fani M, Del Pozzo L, Abiraj K, et al. PET of somatostatin receptor-positive tumors using ^{64}Cu- and ^{68}Ga-somatostatin antagonists: the chelate makes the difference. J Nucl Med 2011;52:1110–8.

56. Ginj M, Zhang H, Waser B, et al. Radiolabeled somatostatin receptor antagonists are preferable to agonists for in vivo peptide receptor targeting of tumors. Proc Natl Acad Sci U S A 2006;103: 16436–41.

57. Wild D, Fani M, Béhé M, et al. First clinical evidence that imaging with somatostatin receptor antagonists is feasible. J Nucl Med 2011;52:1412–7.

58. Wild D, Fani M, Fischer R, et al. Comparison of somatostatin receptor agonist and antagonist for peptide receptor radionuclide therapy: a pilot study. J Nucl Med 2014;55:1248–52.

59. de Castiglione R, Gozzini L. Bombesin receptor antagonists. Crit Rev Oncol Hematol 1996;24:117–51.

60. Stangelberger A, Schally AV, Varga JL, et al. Inhibition of human androgen-independent PC-3 and DU-145 prostate cancers by antagonists of bombesin and growth hormone releasing hormone is linked to PKC, MAPK and c-jun intracellular signalling. Eur J Cancer 2005;41:2735–44.

61. Heinrich E, Schally AV, Buchholz S, et al. Dose-dependent growth inhibition in vivo of PC-3 prostate cancer with a reduction in tumoral growth factors after therapy with GHRH antagonist MZ-J-7-138. Prostate 2008;68:1763–72.

62. Miyazaki M, Lamharzi N, Schally AV, et al. Inhibition of growth of MDA-MB-231 human breast cancer xenografts in nude mice by bombesin/gastrin-releasing peptide (GRP) antagonists RC-3940-II and RC-3095. Eur J Cancer 1998;34:710–7.

63. Bajo AM, Schally AV, Groot K, et al. Bombesin antagonists inhibit proangiogenic factors in human experimental breast cancers. Br J Cancer 2004; 90:245–52.

64. Moody TW, Mantey SA, Pradhan TK, et al. Development of high affinity camptothecin-bombesin conjugates that have targeted cytotoxicity for bombesin receptor-containing tumor cells. J Biol Chem 2004; 279:23580–9.

65. Kanashiro CA, Schally AV, Groot K, et al. Inhibition of mutant p53 expression and growth of DMS-153 small cell lung carcinoma by antagonists of growth hormone-releasing hormone and bombesin. Proc Natl Acad Sci U S A 2003;100:15836–41.

66. Szereday Z, Schally AV, Varga JL, et al. Antagonists of growth hormone-releasing hormone inhibit the proliferation of experimental non-small cell lung carcinoma. Cancer Res 2003;63:7913–9.

67. Martinez J, Rodriguez M, Bali JP, et al. Phenylethylamide derivatives of the C-terminal tetrapeptide of gastrin. Potent inhibitors of gastrin-stimulated acid secretion. Int J Pept Protein Res 1986;28:529–35.

68. Martinez J, Rodriguez M, Bali JP, et al. Phenethyl ester derivative analogues of the C-terminal tetrapeptide of gastrin as potent gastrin antagonists. J Med Chem 1986;29:2201–6.

69. Wang LH, Coy DH, Taylor JE, et al. des-Met carboxyl-terminally modified analogues of bombesin function as potent bombesin receptor antagonists, partial agonists, or agonists. J Biol Chem 1990;265:15695–703.

70. Wang LH, Coy DH, Taylor JE, et al. Desmethionine alkylamide bombesin analogues: a new class of bombesin receptor antagonists with potent antisecretory activity in pancreatic acini and antimitotic activity in Swiss 3T3 cells. Biochemistry 1990;29: 616–22.

71. Davis TP, Crowell S, Taylor J, et al. Metabolic stability and tumor inhibition of bombesin/GRP receptor antagonists. Peptides 1992;13:401–7.

72. Nock B, Nikolopoulou A, Chiotellis E, et al. [99mTc] Demobesin 1, a novel potent bombesin analogue for GRP receptor-targeted tumour imaging. Eur J Nucl Med Mol Imaging 2003;30:247–58.

73. Breeman WA, Hofland LJ, de Jong M, et al. Evaluation of radiolabelled bombesin analogues for receptor-targeted scintigraphy and radiotherapy. Int J Cancer 1999;81:658–65.

74. Maina T, Bergsma H, Kulkarni HR, et al. Preclinical and first clinical experience with the gastrin-releasing peptide receptor-antagonist [68Ga]SB3 and PET/CT. Eur J Nucl Med Mol Imaging 2016;43:964–73.

75. Bakker IL, Fröberg AC, Busstra M, et al. PET imaging of therapy-naïve primary prostate cancer patients using the GRPr-targeting ligand Sarabesin 3. Eur Urol Suppl 2016;15(3):e567.

76. Lymperis E, Maina T, Kaloudi A, et al. Transient in vivo NEP inhibition enhances the theranostic potential of the new GRPR-antagonist [111In/177Lu] SB3. Eur J Nucl Med Mol Imaging 2014;41:S319.

77. Shipp MA, Tarr GE, Chen CY, et al. CD10/neutral endopeptidase 24.11 hydrolyzes bombesin-like peptides and regulates the growth of small cell carcinomas of the lung. Proc Natl Acad Sci U S A 1991;88:10662–6.

78. Linder KE, Metcalfe E, Arunachalam T, et al. In vitro and in vivo metabolism of Lu-AMBA, a GRP-receptor binding compound, and the synthesis and characterization of its metabolites. Bioconjug Chem 2009;20: 1171–8.

79. Nock BA, Maina T, Krenning EP, et al. "To serve and protect": enzyme inhibitors as radiopeptide escorts promote tumor targeting. J Nucl Med 2014;55:121–7.

80. Abd-Elgaliel WR, Gallazzi F, Garrison JC, et al. Design, synthesis, and biological evaluation of an antagonist-bombesin analogue as targeting vector. Bioconjug Chem 2008;19:2040–8.

81. Azay J, Nagain C, Llinares M, et al. Comparative study of in vitro and in vivo activities of bombesin pseudopeptide analogs modified on the C-terminal dipeptide fragment. Peptides 1998;19:57–63.

82. Tokita K, Katsuno T, Hocart SJ, et al. Molecular basis for selectivity of high affinity peptide antagonists for the gastrin-releasing peptide receptor. J Biol Chem 2001;276:36652–63.

83. Gourni E, Mansi R, Jamous M, et al. N-terminal modifications improve the receptor affinity and pharmacokinetics of radiolabeled peptidic gastrin-releasing peptide receptor antagonists: examples of 68Ga- and 64Cu-labeled peptides for PET imaging. J Nucl Med 2014;55:1719–25.

84. Abiraj K, Mansi R, Tamma ML, et al. Bombesin antagonist-based radioligands for translational nuclear imaging of gastrin-releasing peptide receptor-positive tumors. J Nucl Med 2011;52:1970–8.

85. Varasteh Z, Rosenstrom U, Velikyan I, et al. The effect of mini-PEG-based spacer length on binding and pharmacokinetic properties of a 68Ga-labeled NOTA-conjugated antagonistic analog of bombesin. Molecules 2014;19:10455–72.

86. Varasteh Z, Mitran B, Rosenstrom U, et al. The effect of macrocyclic chelators on the targeting properties of the 68Ga-labeled gastrin releasing peptide receptor antagonist PEG2-RM26. Nucl Med Biol 2015;42:446–54.

87. Mitran B, Varasteh Z, Selvaraju RK, et al. Selection of optimal chelator improves the contrast of GRPR imaging using bombesin analogue RM26. Int J Oncol 2016;48:2124–34.

88. Mansi R, Wang X, Forrer F, et al. Evaluation of a 1,4,7,10-tetraazacyclododecane-1,4,7,10-tetraacetic acid-conjugated bombesin-based radioantagonist for the labeling with single-photon emission computed tomography, positron emission tomography, and therapeutic radionuclides. Clin Cancer Res 2009;15:5240–9.

89. Marsouvanidis PJ, Nock BA, Hajjaj B, et al. Gastrin releasing peptide receptor-directed radioligands based on a bombesin antagonist: synthesis, ^{111}In-labeling, and preclinical profile. J Med Chem 2013; 56:2374–84.

90. Abiraj K, Mansi R, Tamma ML, et al. Tetraamine-derived bifunctional chelators for technetium-99m labelling: synthesis, bioconjugation and evaluation as targeted SPECT imaging probes for GRP-receptor-positive tumours. Chemistry 2010;16: 2115–24.

91. Dumont RA, Tamma M, Braun F, et al. Targeted radiotherapy of prostate cancer with a gastrin-releasing peptide receptor antagonist is effective as monotherapy and in combination with rapamycin. J Nucl Med 2013;54:762–9.

92. Chatalic KL, Konijnenberg M, Nonnekens J, et al. In vivo stabilization of a gastrin-releasing peptide receptor antagonist enhances PET imaging and radionuclide therapy of prostate cancer in preclinical studies. Theranostics 2016;6:104–17.

93. Kim K, Zhang H, LaRosa S, et al. Bombesin antagonist based radiotherapy of prostate cancer combined with WST-11 vascular targeted photodynamic therapy. Clin Cancer Res 2017. http://dx.doi.org/10.1158/1078-0432.CCR-16-2745. [Epub ahead of print].

94. Jamous M, Tamma ML, Gourni E, et al. PEG spacers of different length influence the biological profile of bombesin-based radiolabeled antagonists. Nucl Med Biol 2014;41:464–70.

95. Mansi R, Wang X, Forrer F, et al. Development of a potent DOTA-conjugated bombesin antagonist for targeting GRPr-positive tumours. Eur J Nucl Med Mol Imaging 2011;38:97–107.

96. Nock B, Maina T. Tetraamine-coupled peptides and resulting ^{99m}Tc-radioligands: an effective route for receptor-targeted diagnostic imaging of human tumors. Curr Top Med Chem 2012;12: 2655–67.

97. Kähkönen E, Jambor I, Kemppainen J, et al. In vivo imaging of prostate cancer using [68Ga]-labeled bombesin analog BAY86-7548. Clin Cancer Res 2013;19:5434–43.

98. Minamimoto R, Hancock S, Schneider B, et al. Pilot comparison of ^{68}Ga-RM2 PET and ^{68}Ga-PSMA-11 PET in patients with biochemically recurrent prostate cancer. J Nucl Med 2016;57:557–62.

99. Afshar-Oromieh A, Avtzi E, Giesel FL, et al. The diagnostic value of PET/CT imaging with the ^{68}Ga-labelled PSMA ligand HBED-CC in the diagnosis of recurrent prostate cancer. Eur J Nucl Med Mol Imaging 2015;42:197–209.

100. Guba M, Koehl GE, Neppl E, et al. Dosing of rapamycin is critical to achieve an optimal antiangiogenic effect against cancer. Transpl Int 2005;18:89–94.

101. Popp I, Del Pozzo L, Waser B, et al. Approaches to improve metabolic stability of a statine-based GRP receptor antagonist. Nucl Med Biol 2016;45:22–9.

102. Roivainen A, Kähkönen E, Luoto P, et al. Plasma pharmacokinetics, whole-body distribution, metabolism, and radiation dosimetry of ^{68}Ga bombesin antagonist BAY 86-7548 in healthy men. J Nucl Med 2013;54:867–72.

103. Martinez A, Martinez-Ramirez M, Martinez-Caballero D, et al. Radioimmunotherapy for non-Hodgkin's lymphoma; positioning, safety, and efficacy of ^{90}Y-Ibritumomab. 10 years of experience and follow-up. Rev Esp Med Nucl Imagen Mol 2017;36: 13–9.

104. Seregni E, Maccauro M, Chiesa C, et al. Treatment with tandem ^{90}Y]DOTA-TATE and ^{177}Lu]DOTA-TATE of neuroendocrine tumours refractory to conventional therapy. Eur J Nucl Med Mol Imaging 2014;41:223–30.

105. Marincek N, Jorg AC, Brunner P, et al. Somatostatin-based radiotherapy with ^{90}Y-DOTA]-TOC in neuroendocrine tumors: long-term outcome of a phase I dose escalation study. J Transl Med 2013;11:17.

106. Lohrmann C, Zhang H, Thorek DL, et al. Cerenkov luminescence imaging for radiation dose calculation of a ^{90}Y-labeled gastrin-releasing peptide receptor antagonist. J Nucl Med 2015;56:805–11.

107. Wieser G, Mansi R, Grosu AL, et al. Positron emission tomography (PET) imaging of prostate cancer with a gastrin releasing peptide receptor antagonist–from mice to men. Theranostics 2014;4:412–9.

108. Heimbrook DC, Saari WS, Balishin NL, et al. Gastrin releasing peptide antagonists with improved potency and stability. J Med Chem 1991;34:2102–7.

109. Nock BA, Kaloudi A, Lymperis E, et al. Theranostic perspectives in prostate cancer with the gastrin-releasing peptide receptor antagonist NeoBOMB1: preclinical and first clinical results. J Nucl Med 2017;58:75–80.

110. Maina T, Kaloudi A, Giarika A, et al. [68Ga]NeoBOMB1, a new candidate in the diagnosis of breast cancer: first results in GRPR-expressing cells and animal models. Eur J Nucl Med Mol Imaging 2016;43(Suppl 1):S104.

111. Dalm SU, Bakker IL, de Blois E, et al. [68]Ga/^{177}Lu-NeoBOMB1, a novel radiolabeled GRPR antagonist for theranostic use in oncology. J Nucl Med 2017;58(2):293–9.

112. Paulmichl A, Summer D, Manzl C, et al. Targeting gastrointestinal stromal tumor with ^{68}Ga-labeled

peptides: an in vitro study on gastrointestinal stromal tumor-cell lines. Cancer Biother Radiopharm 2016;31:302–10.

113. Baum RP, Kulkarni HR. THERANOSTICS: from molecular imaging using Ga-68 labeled tracers and PET/CT to personalized radionuclide therapy - the Bad Berka experience. Theranostics 2012;2: 437–47.

114. Kulkarni HR, Singh A, Schuchardt C, et al. PSMA-Based radioligand therapy for metastatic castration-resistant prostate cancer: the Bad Berka

experience since 2013. J Nucl Med 2016;57: 97S–104S.

115. Baum RP, Kulkarni HR, Schuchardt C, et al. ^{177}Lu-Labeled prostate-specific membrane antigen radioligand therapy of metastatic castration-resistant prostate cancer: safety and efficacy. J Nucl Med 2016;57:1006–13.

116. Meckel M, Nauth A, Timpe J, et al. Development of a ^{177}Lu]BPAMD labeling kit and an automated synthesis module for routine bone targeted endoradiotherapy. Cancer Biother Radiopharm 2015;30:94–9.

Urokinase Plasminogen Activator Receptor–PET with ^{68}Ga-NOTA-AE105
First Clinical Experience with a Novel PET Ligand

Dorthe Skovgaard, MD, PhD[a], Morten Persson, MSc, PhD[b],
Andreas Kjaer, MD, PhD, DMSc[a],*

KEYWORDS

- PET • Oncology • Prostate cancer • Breast cancer • Theranostics • Molecular imaging
- Invasiveness • Prognostication

KEY POINTS

- Urokinase plasminogen activator receptor (uPAR) is a key component in proteolysis and extracellular matrix degradation during cancer invasion and metastasis.
- uPAR expression in several types of cancer provides independent prognostic information.
- PET imaging of uPAR with ^{68}Ga-NOTA-AE105 is a new and clinically relevant diagnostic and prognostic biomarker.
- A first-in-human PET study with the novel ligand ^{68}Ga-NOTA-AE105, including patients with prostate, breast, and urinary bladder cancer, has shown encouraging data that support large-scale clinical trials.

INTRODUCTION

Diagnostic molecular imaging techniques are gaining importance as the therapeutic paradigm changes from clinical decisions based on morphologic tumor detection only to the ability to distinguish patients with indolent tumors that can be managed conservatively, from patients with more aggressive tumors that may require immediate treatment with surgery, intensive chemotherapy regimens or radiation therapy.[1] This has led to a search for upregulated tumor-specific markers that can serve as candidates for tumor imaging with the potential of identifying the aggressive tumor phenotype.[2] Metastasis formation is one of the "hallmarks of cancer," and it is the ability of the cancer cells to invade the surrounding stromal tissue and form distant metastases that leads to progression and poor prognosis.[3] Recently, a series of promising preclinical PET imaging studies

Disclosure Statement: A. Kjaer and M. Persson are inventors of the composition of matter of uPAR PET with a filed patent application: *Positron Emitting Radionuclides Labeled Peptides for Human uPAR PET Imaging* (WO 2014/086364 A1). M. Persson and A. Kjaer are cofounders of Curasight that has licensed the uPAR PET patent to commercialize uPAR PET technology. D. Skovgaard has received funding from Curasight and participates in research involving ^{68}Ga-NOTA-AE105.
[a] Department of Clinical Physiology, Nuclear Medicine & PET, Cluster for Molecular Imaging Rigshospitalet and University of Copenhagen, Blegdamsvej 9, 4011, Copenhagen DK-2100, Denmark; [b] Curasight, Ole Maaloesvej 3, Copenhagen DK-2200, Denmark
* Corresponding author.
E-mail address: akjaer@sund.ku.dk

PET Clin 12 (2017) 311–319
http://dx.doi.org/10.1016/j.cpet.2017.02.003
1556-8598/17/© 2017 Elsevier Inc. All rights reserved.

in rodent cancer models and clinical translation of the novel PET ligand ^{68}Ga-NOTA-AE105[4] hold promise to provide the first noninvasive imaging of the metastatic process by targeting the important urokinase plasminogen activator system.

BIOLOGY OF THE UROKINASE PLASMINOGEN ACTIVATOR SYSTEM

Numerous studies have implicated the serine-protease urokinase-type plasminogen activator (uPA) and its receptor (uPAR) to be of special importance in cancer invasion and metastasis.[5–9] uPAR is a receptor consisting of 3 domains (DI, DII, DIII) bound to the cell surface via a glycolipid-anchor.[10,11] uPA binds with high affinity to uPAR and consequently converts plasminogen to active plasmin, which activates several proteases related to the proteolytic degradation of extracellular matrix, thereby facilitating cancer cell invasion (**Fig. 1**). In addition, uPA/uPAR directly influences multiple other aspects of tumor progression and development by eliciting tumor-associated processes, such as cell proliferation, cell adhesion and migration, chemotaxis, and cell survival through interactions with coreceptors to affect intracellular downstream signaling.[12] In clinical studies, uPAR has significant prognostic information in cancers, such as breast, lung, colorectal, and prostate, in which patients with high levels of cleaved uPAR that form in the blood experience a shorter overall survival.[13–15] Using various biochemical assays, immunohistochemistry (IHC), tissue micro-arrays, and reverse transcriptase-polymerase chain reaction (PCR), uPAR expression also can be assessed directly in tumor specimens. High expression levels of uPAR in tumors have indeed shown a strong association with metastatic disease, and shorter progression-free survival and overall survival. Importantly, the expression of uPAR is very low or undetectable in normal non-cancer, homeostatic tissues, which would translate to a favorable tumor-to-background ratio when used for imaging purposes.[16–18] All these characteristics, including that uPAR is a glycosyl phosphatidylinositol (GPI)-anchored receptor attached to the outside surface of the cell membrane,[19] make uPAR a potential ideal target for both imaging and therapy for improved diagnosing, risk stratification, and treatment monitoring, as also suggested by others.[20,21]

PRESENCE AND SIGNIFICANCE OF UROKINASE PLASMINOGEN ACTIVATOR RECEPTOR IN SELECTED TUMORS

uPAR as an imaging target seems promising in multiple cancer types due to the well-documented expression pattern of uPAR in nearly all cancer indications.[13,16,17] However, in this review we have chosen to describe the differential distribution and the physiologic and pathologic role of uPAR, with emphasis on 5 cancer types in which uPAR seem to be of most obvious potential. This includes breast, prostate, urinary bladder, and pancreatic cancer and glioblastoma. Common for all 5 types of cancer, besides documented high expression levels of uPAR, is that PET with fluodeoxyglucose (FDG-PET) imaging in diagnostic and preoperative

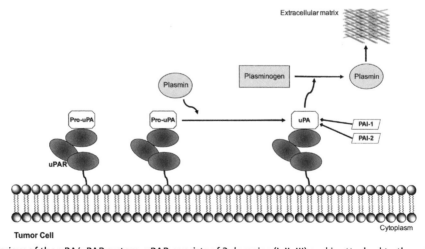

Fig. 1. Overview of the uPA/uPAR system. uPAR consists of 3 domains (I, II, III) and is attached to the cell surface by a GPI anchor. uPA bound to uPAR cleaves plasminogen, generating the active protease plasmin. uPAR-bound pro-uPA is also activated by plasmin, which in turn results in a feedback pathway that accelerates plasminogen activation. Plasmin activates matrix metalloproteases (MMPs). Both plasmin and MMPs degrade extracellular matrix and thereby promote cancer invasion and metastasis. Proteolytic activities of uPA and plasmin are inhibited by plasminogen activator inhibitor (PAI)-1 and PAI-2.

workup has been shown to be of limited value or is not routinely recommended.[22,23] As a result of this, there is an unmet clinical need to develop new imaging ligands with superior specificity and sensitivity, giving patients with these specific types of cancers the potential benefit of the combination of anatomic and molecular imaging with PET/computed tomography (CT). An important notion is that uPAR is not only expressed on tumor cells but also largely present in the immediate tumor-surrounding stroma. Static PET imaging cannot distinguish the origin of the signal. However, that is not perceived as a problem for the utility of uPAR PET, because uPAR expression in the cancer-associated stromal cells confers substantially to the overall uPAR content in various tumor types and therefore contributes significantly to the achievable prognostic information.[24,25]

Breast Cancer

Breast cancer was the first cancer disease in which prognosis was shown to be associated with the plasminogen activator system. Accordingly, high levels of uPAR in patients with breast cancer are linked to shorter regression-free survival, overall survival, and prediction of treatment resistance in multiple studies.[26–28] In addition, high levels of uPAR expression have been documented in triple-negative breast cancer, tamoxifen-refractory breast cancer, and in a subset of HER2-positive breast tumors, all of which are classified as aggressive.[29] In breast tumor tissue, uPAR immunoreactivity is mainly located in the stromal compartment, where especially macrophages surrounding the malignant epithelium contain high expression levels of uPAR.[26,30] As an important prerequisite for uPAR imaging of breast cancer, only 2% of patients have uPAR levels below the detection limit.[26]

Prostate Cancer

In prostate cancer, uPAR levels in both plasma (termed soluble uPAR or suPAR) and in tumor tissue are associated with relevant pathologic and clinical parameters such as high Gleason score, advanced tumor stage, lymph node metastases, shorter recurrence-free and overall survival.[31] uPAR immunostaining of tumor tissue samples has revealed uPAR to be located mainly on neutrophils and macrophages surrounding the cancer cells.[32] One of the major challenges when assessing uPAR expression directly in tumor specimen is intratumor heterogeneity.[33] This is of special importance in prostate cancer, which is recognized as being a multifocal disease with a broad spectrum of clinical, pathologic, and molecular characteristics, emphasized by the routinely used

12-core biopsy protocol for diagnosis of prostate cancer.[34] uPAR PET offers an attractive method that can provide the required quantitative information on the uPAR expression profile, without the need for invasive procedures and the risk of missing the target, that is, *sampling error*, due to tumor heterogeneity.

Urinary Bladder Cancer

Urinary bladder tumors account for 90% to 95% of the urothelial carcinomas and are the most common malignancy of the urinary tract. Although most patients with bladder cancer are diagnosed with non–muscle-invasive disease, approximately 20% to 40% of patients either present with or subsequently develop more advanced disease.[35] Elevated urinary levels of uPA and uPAR have been found in patients with bladder carcinoma compared with urinary levels of healthy controls.[36] Importantly, uPA/uPAR expression in tumor lesions and the plasma level of uPA/uPAR give additional independent prognostic information.[37–42] In a recent study in which uPAR positivity by immunostaining was found in 122 (89%) of 137 and 118 (74%) of 149 cases at the invasive front and tumor core, respectively, uPAR expression was primarily expressed by myofibroblasts and macrophages in the surrounding stroma as well as in some cancer cells.[41]

Glioblastoma

In glioblastoma, uPAR expression also has been reported elevated and to correlate with parenchymal invasion; that is, aggressiveness.[43–45] uPAR has been found to be localized to astrocytoma cells and endothelial cells within tumor tissue, especially near sites of vascular proliferation and at the leading edges of tumors. Very low expression has been reported in low-grade astrocytomas and normal brain tissues, thus underscoring the promising potential of uPAR as imaging target for glioblastoma, as also recognized by others.[46] Further, a recent study has provided evidence for a direct link between upregulation of the uPA-uPAR-ERK1/2 pathway and sensitivity toward small molecule tyrosine kinase inhibitors for the epidermal growth factor receptor (EGFR).[47] Together, this makes uPAR a highly promising imaging target for gliomas, with the potential of diagnosis/risk stratification and as a tool for identification of patients sensitive to EGFR inhibitors.

Pancreatic Cancer

Pancreatic cancer has an extremely poor prognosis; the median survival time for all patients is 4 to 6 months, and the overall 5-year survival rate is 7.2%.[48] Emerging evidence suggest that uPA and uPAR are significant in pancreatic cancer invasion and metastasis.[49–51] Most pancreatic adeno-carcinomas express uPAR, and overexpression of uPAR in one study was found in 48 of 50 invasive carcinomas, as well as in a large proportion of high-grade pancreatic cancer lesions by immunohistochemistry and in situ hybridization.[52] In line with other cancers, the overexpression of uPAR in pancreatic cancer also has been found to be a strong and independent predictor of short overall survival.[53]

UROKINASE PLASMINOGEN ACTIVATOR RECEPTOR–PET IMAGING: PRECLINICAL STUDIES

In a large series of peptides, the linear 9 amino acid peptide, denoted AE105 (Asp-Cha-Phe-D-Ser-D-Arg-Tyr-Leu-Trp-Ser), was originally identified by affinity maturation using combinatorial chemistry to bind with high affinity to human uPAR.[54] AE105 forms a tight 1:1 complex with purified uPAR, displaying a K_D of 0.4 nM with a k_{off} of 2×10 to $4 \ s^{-1}$ as measured by surface plasmon resonance. Furthermore, AE105 is a potent competitive inhibitor of the uPA•uPAR interaction displaying a half

maximal inhibitory concentration value of approximately 11 nM in a purified system.[54] Furthermore, the binding pocket of AE105 for uPAR has been elucidated and studies have revealed that modifications in the N-terminal can be done without losing binding affinity.[55] Based on this, multiple uPAR-targeted PET ligands based on AE105 using different bifunctional chelators and PET isotopes have been generated and investigated in various human cancer mouse models.[55–59]

One particularly interesting version is based on the NOTA-chelator conjugated in the N-terminal (eg, NOTA-AE105). This peptide conjugate was labeled with Al[18]F as the first example of a fluorine-18 (^{18}F)-labeled uPAR-targeting PET ligand.[58] The promising proof-of-concept results that were found by using this uPAR PET ligand in a human prostate cancer mouse model let us pursue the development of a gallium-68 (^{68}Ga)-labeled version. The main advantage for using ^{68}Ga instead of Al[18]F is that ^{68}Ga is generator-based compared with the Al[18]F, which needs a cyclotron; thus, the potential future clinical availability of uPAR PET can be dramatically increased.

The synthesis and the first evidence of the usefulness for glioblastoma imaging of ^{68}Ga-NOTA-AE105, was recently provided (**Fig. 2**).[60] In that study,

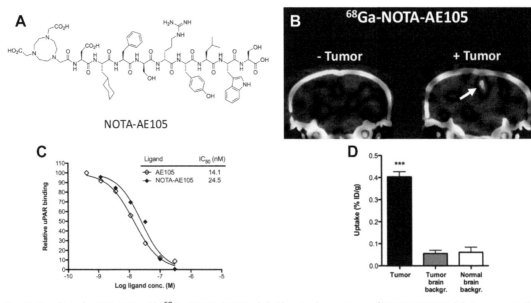

Fig. 2. Preclinical uPAR PET with ^{68}Ga-NOTA-AE105. (A) Chemical structure of NOTA-AE105. (B) Representative coronal PET images of a mouse with an orthotopic patient-derived glioblastoma tumor (+Tumor, *white arrows*) and a normal mouse with tumor (−Tumor) following ^{68}Ga-NOTA-AE105 injection. (C) In vitro competitive inhibition of the uPA:uPAR binding for AE105 and NOTA-AE105. The interactions of AE105 and NOTA-AE105 (see **Fig. 1**) with immobilized human uPAR were measured in real time by surface plasmon resonance. A small reduction in the efficacy to compete the uPA•uPAR interaction because of the NOTA conjugation was found (AE105: IC50, 14.1 nM, vs NOTA-AE105: IC50, 24.5 nM). (D) Quantitative uptake in tumor (Tumor), hemisphere contralateral to tumor (Tumor brain), and normal brain with no tumor (Normal brain), 1 hour after injection of ^{68}Ga-NOTA-AE105. ***P<.001 versus brain background.

an orthotopic glioblastoma model was used to demonstrate strong accumulation of ^{68}Ga-NOTA-AE105 in the tumor and compared with the amino acid tracer ^{18}F-fluoroethyltyrosine (^{18}F-FET). ^{68}Ga-NOTA-AE105 showed lower absolute uptake values but higher tumor-to-background ratios. However, a strong species selectivity was seen for the interaction of human uPAR and AE105, as no measurable competition of the orthologous mouse uPA●uPAR interaction was observed,[61] which underscores that all preclinical study results with this system should be interpreted with caution. Nevertheless, subsequent autoradiography on resected tumor tissue revealed intratumoral tracer distribution, which resembled the immunohistochemical staining of uPAR, thus providing strong evidence for uPAR specificity of ^{68}Ga-NOTA-AE105.

CLINICAL EXPERIENCES

Based on the promising preclinical studies, the *first-in-humans* trial of ^{68}Ga-NOTA-AE105 was recently conducted (ClinicalTrials.gov: NCT02437539).[4] By definition, the primary endpoints of a phase I clinical study are safety, biodistribution, and dosimetry assessment. The study included 10 patients with cancer with 3 different solid tumors: urinary bladder (2 patients), breast (2 patients), and prostate cancer (6 patients). The biodistribution and radiation dosimetry were assessed by serial whole-body PET/CT scans (at 10 minutes, and 1 and 2 hours postinjection). Importantly, no adverse events or clinically detectable pharmacologic effects were found. Radiation dosimetry analysis revealed an effective

dose of 0.0276 mSv/MBq, being in the same range as a routine FDG-PET.[62] The bladder was the organ with the highest absorbed dose (0.131 mGy/MBq), followed by the kidneys (0.070 mGy/MBq), corresponding to a main excretion route through the kidneys. Plasma pharmacokinetic and urine metabolite analysis revealed intact ^{68}Ga-NOTA-AE105 in blood and urine with no formation of isotopic-labeled metabolites and a plasma half-life of 8.5 minutes. Persistently, there was a relatively high, but decreasing blood pool activity that probably reflects plasma protein–bound activity.

Importantly, this phase I study also provided the first preliminary clinical experience with ^{68}Ga-NOTA-AE105 uptake in primary tumor lesions and metastases. uPAR PET with ^{68}Ga-NOTA-AE105 provided satisfactory image contrast and identification of primary tumors and metastases with a heterogeneous intralesional uptake pattern and moderate variability within tumors, as expected due to differential cellular expression of uPAR in malignant tissue. Maximal standardized uptake values (SUV$_{max}$) in primary tumor lesions varied from 3.7 to 5.1 (at 10 minutes postinjection). Two patients with newly diagnosed breast cancer were included before surgical intervention with lumpectomy and complete axillary lymph node dissection. PET with ^{68}Ga-NOTA-AE105 clearly visualized the primary tumors and metastatic spread to the ipsilateral axillary lymph nodes in both patients. Interestingly, in one of these patients, the metastatic spread was not found on the routine preoperative diagnostic workup with ultrasound and fine-needle biopsy (**Fig. 3**). Accordingly, ^{68}Ga-NOTA-AE105 PET could

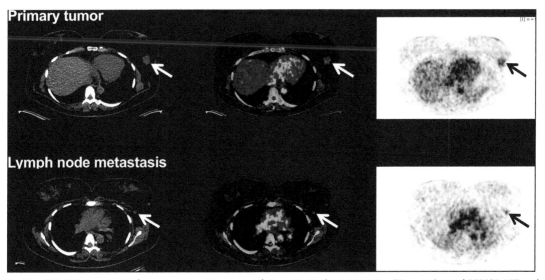

Fig. 3. uPAR PET imaging in breast cancer. *Upper panel*: Representative transverse CT, coregistered PET/CT, PET and images of a primary tumor lesion (*arrows*) with intense uptake of ^{68}Ga-NOTA-AE105. *Lower panel*: Images show a uPAR PET-positive axillary lymph node metastasis (*arrows*) with significant uptake in the same patient. The metastatic spread was not identified at the routine preoperative diagnostic workup with ultrasound and fine-needle biopsy.

have higher sensitivity in detecting lymph node metastases than the current preoperative diagnostic workup. uPAR immunohistochemistry on surgical specimens of primary tumors and metastatic lymph nodes in both patients confirmed positive uPAR expression.

Six patients with prostate cancer were included, ranging from patients with newly diagnosed locally advanced disease to patients with disseminated prostate cancer and multiple bone metastases. In patients with locally advanced prostate cancer (4 patients), ^{68}Ga-NOTA-AE105 exhibited a low, heterogeneous intraprostatic distribution of the radioligand. In contrast, the 2 patients with disseminated prostate cancer had multiple bone metastases with clear and significant ^{68}Ga-NOTA-AE105 uptake, as well as a heterogeneous uptake at the site of the primary tumor within the prostate gland (**Fig. 4**). In addition, 2 patients with urinary bladder cancer were included in the study during an ongoing chemotherapy regimen with only a small amount of residual disease. Both patients had proven response to chemotherapy, as evaluated by routine CT scans, before inclusion in the present study. No clear uptake was seen on these patients, probably because of response to therapy.

Concluding on these preliminary clinical data: uPAR PET shows perceivable, heterogeneous uptake of the ^{68}Ga-NOTA-AE105 in breast and prostate cancer, including primary tumors and lymph node and bone metastases, possibly reflecting relevant disparate uPAR expression patterns. The ability of ^{68}Ga-NOTA-AE105 to image urinary bladder cancer remains to be proven and is currently being investigated. A potential interpretational challenge in uPAR PET in urinary tract malignancies could be urinary excretion of the ligand. Delayed imaging following forced diuresis and oral hydration might be necessary.

FUTURE DIRECTIONS

PET imaging of uPAR expression with ^{68}Ga-NOTA-AE105 seems to be highly promising, and several important clinical questions in both primary and metastatic cancer can potentially be addressed using uPAR PET. An important clinical implication of uPAR PET is preoperative staging. We are currently investigating the ability of uPAR PET to preoperatively identify regional lymph node involvement in breast cancer (Clinicaltrials.gov: NCT02681640) and urinary bladder cancer (Clinicaltrials.gov: NCT02805608). In addition, uPAR PET can possibly be applied in a situation in which initial therapy fails and a relapse is suspected. An example of this could be in the context of biochemical recurrence in prostate cancer, in which relapse is usually initially detected as a rise in serum prostate-specific antigen (PSA) level. In these patients, a sensitive and reliable imaging assessment for localization of the site of recurrent disease would potentially be beneficial in providing high-quality, representative biopsy samples.[63,64]

UROKINASE PLASMINOGEN ACTIVATOR RECEPTOR–PET AS COMPANION DIAGNOSTIC

In addition to imaging, uPAR is a promising candidate as a molecular target for cancer therapy. Several new and specific pharmaceuticals targeting

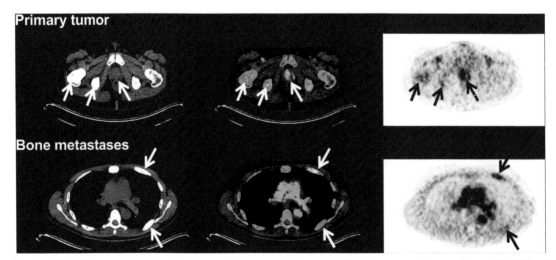

Fig. 4. uPAR PET imaging in prostate cancer. *Upper panel*: Representative transverse CT, coregistered PET/CT and PET images with uptake of ^{68}Ga-NOTA-AE105 at the site of the primary tumor (*right arrow*). In addition, the patient has uPAR PET-positive metastases in right femoral head/neck and ischiadic bone (*left arrows*). *Lower panel*: Images show uPAR PET-positive metastases in costae (*arrows*) with significant uptake in the same patient.

uPAR, including inhibitory recombinant proteins, monoclonal antibodies, protease-activated pro-drugs, and synthetic antagonist peptides, have been investigated.[65] Recently, targeting of uPAR with a monoclonal antibody (ATN-658) blocking the biologic functions of uPAR was shown to have a potent and encouraging therapeutic effect in murine prostate cancer models, including bone metastases formation,[66] and is expected to move into human clinical trial. A noninvasive method for specific assessment of tumor uPAR expression status would be valuable. Such a tool would be clinically relevant for guidance of patient management and as *companion diagnostics* for emerging uPAR-targeting therapies. Importantly, uPAR PET allows assessment of the entire disease burden and avoids sampling errors from biopsies when uPAR expression is heterogeneous.

UROKINASE PLASMINOGEN ACTIVATOR RECEPTOR–PET AS PART OF THERANOSTICS

Another innovative and interesting perspective is to combine noninvasive PET imaging and targeted radionuclide therapy ("theranostics"). Here, the same targeting ligand is radiolabeled with either a positron-emitting nuclide for PET imaging or an alpha/beta emitter nuclide for therapeutic intervention. Such a dual functionality aligns excellently with the concept of *precision medicine*.[67] Targeted radiotherapy has shown promising results in several cancers, with somatostatin receptor–based targeting of neuroendocrine tumors being the most successful so far.[68] In fact, we have conducted 2 preclinical *proof-of-concept* studies with DOTA-AE105 conjugated with the beta emitter ^{177}Lu for uPAR-targeted radionuclide therapy in colorectal cancer[69] and in metastatic prostate cancer.[67] In these preclinical studies, we found a significant reduction in tumor size (colorectal cancer), and fewer metastatic lesions and longer overall metastatic-free survival (prostate cancer) in mice treated with ^{177}Lu-DOTA-AE105 compared with controls, thus setting the stage for a uPAR-mediated theranostic approach.

SUMMARY

uPAR is of major importance in cancer invasion and metastatic development. Therefore, PET imaging of uPAR with the novel ligand ^{68}Ga-NOTA-AE105 has the possibility to become a clinically relevant diagnostic and prognostic imaging biomarker. The first clinical experience with ^{68}Ga-NOTA-AE105 is most encouraging, and several large-scale clinical trials are ongoing and planned to determine the utility of uPAR PET for diagnosing and therapy planning in several forms of cancer.

REFERENCES

1. Weissleder R. Molecular imaging in cancer. Science 2006;312(5777):1168–71.
2. Winnard PT Jr, Pathak AP, Dhara S, et al. Molecular imaging of metastatic potential. J Nucl Med 2008; 49(Suppl 2):96S–112S.
3. Hanahan D, Weinberg RA. Hallmarks of cancer: the next generation. Cell. 2011;144(5):646–74.
4. Skovgaard D, Persson M, Brandt-Larsen M, et al. Safety, dosimetry, and tumor detection ability of (68)Ga-NOTA-AE105: first-in-human study of a novel radioligand for uPAR PET imaging. J Nucl Med 2017;58(3):379–86.
5. Sporn MB. The war on cancer. Lancet 1996;347(9012): 1377–81.
6. Dano K, Behrendt N, Hoyer-Hansen G, et al. Plasminogen activation and cancer. Thromb Haemost 2005;93(4):676–81.
7. Jacobsen B, Ploug M. The urokinase receptor and its structural homologue C4.4A in human cancer: expression, prognosis and pharmacological inhibition. Curr Med Chem 2008;15(25):2559–73.
8. Dass K, Ahmad A, Azmi AS, et al. Evolving role of uPA/uPAR system in human cancers. Cancer Treat Rev 2008;34(2):122–36.
9. Ulisse S, Baldini E, Sorrenti S, et al. The urokinase plasminogen activator system: a target for anti-cancer therapy. Curr Cancer Drug Targets 2009;9(1):32–71.
10. Llinas P, Le Du MH, Gardsvoll H, et al. Crystal structure of the human urokinase plasminogen activator receptor bound to an antagonist peptide. EMBO J 2005;24(9):1655–63.
11. Kjaergaard M, Hansen LV, Jacobsen B, et al. Structure and ligand interactions of the urokinase receptor (uPAR). Front Biosci 2008;13:5441–61.
12. Blasi F, Sidenius N. The urokinase receptor: focused cell surface proteolysis, cell adhesion and signaling. FEBS Lett 2010;584(9):1923–30.
13. de Bock CE, Wang Y. Clinical significance of urokinase-type plasminogen activator receptor (uPAR) expression in cancer. Med Res Rev 2004;24(1):13–39.
14. Rasch MG, Lund IK, Almasi CE, et al. Intact and cleaved uPAR forms: diagnostic and prognostic value in cancer. Front Biosci 2008;13:6752–62.
15. Boonstra MC, Verspaget HW, Ganesh S, et al. Clinical applications of the urokinase receptor (uPAR) for cancer patients. Curr Pharm Des 2011;17(19): 1890–910.
16. Illemann M, Bird N, Majeed A, et al. Two distinct expression patterns of urokinase, urokinase receptor and plasminogen activator inhibitor-1 in colon cancer liver metastases. Int J Cancer 2009;124(8): 1860–70.

17. Nielsen BS, Rank F, Illemann M, et al. Stromal cells associated with early invasive foci in human mammary ductal carcinoma in situ coexpress urokinase and urokinase receptor. Int J Cancer 2007;120(10): 2086–95.

18. Dublin E, Hanby A, Patel NK, et al. Immunohistochemical expression of uPA, uPAR, and PAI-1 in breast carcinoma. Fibroblastic expression has strong associations with tumor pathology. Am J Pathol 2000;157(4):1219–27.

19. Ploug M, Behrendt N, Lober D, et al. Protein structure and membrane anchorage of the cellular receptor for urokinase-type plasminogen activator. Semin Thromb Hemost 1991;17(3):183–93.

20. Yang Y, Adelstein SJ, Kassis AI. General approach to identifying potential targets for cancer imaging by integrated bioinformatics analysis of publicly available genomic profiles. Mol Imaging 2011; 10(2):123–34.

21. Li D, Liu S, Shan H, et al. Urokinase plasminogen activator receptor (uPAR) targeted nuclear imaging and radionuclide therapy. Theranostics 2013;3(7): 507–15.

22. Fletcher JW, Djulbegovic B, Soares HP, et al. Recommendations on the use of 18F-FDG PET in oncology. J Nucl Med 2008;49(3):480–508.

23. Agrawal A, Rangarajan V. Appropriateness criteria of FDG PET/CT in oncology. Indian J Radiol Imaging 2015;25(2):88–101.

24. Boonstra MC, Verbeek FP, Mazar AP, et al. Expression of uPAR in tumor-associated stromal cells is associated with colorectal cancer patient prognosis: a TMA study. BMC Cancer 2014;14:269.

25. Boonstra MC, van Driel PB, van Willigen DM, et al. uPAR-targeted multimodal tracer for pre- and intraoperative imaging in cancer surgery. Oncotarget 2015;6(16):14260–73.

26. Grondahl-Hansen J, Peters HA, van Putten WL, et al. Prognostic significance of the receptor for urokinase plasminogen activator in breast cancer. Clin Cancer Res 1995;1:1079–87.

27. Foekens JA, Peters HA, Look MP, et al. The urokinase system of plasminogen activation and prognosis in 2780 breast cancer patients. Cancer Res 2000;60(3):636–43.

28. de Witte JH, Foekens JA, Brunner N, et al. Prognostic impact of urokinase-type plasminogen activator receptor (uPAR) in cytosols and pellet extracts derived from primary breast tumours. Br J Cancer 2001;85(1):85–92.

29. LeBeau AM, Sevillano N, King ML, et al. Imaging the urokinase plasminongen activator receptor in preclinical breast cancer models of acquired drug resistance. Theranostics 2014;4(3):267–79.

30. Pyke C, Graem N, Ralfkiaer E, et al. Receptor for urokinase is present in tumor-associated macrophages in ductal breast carcinoma. Cancer Res 1993;53(8): 1911–5.

31. Shariat SF, Roehrborn CG, McConnell JD, et al. Association of the circulating levels of the urokinase system of plasminogen activation with the presence of prostate cancer and invasion, progression, and metastasis. J Clin Oncol 2007;25(4):349–55.

32. Gupta A, Lotan Y, Ashfaq R, et al. Predictive value of the differential expression of the urokinase plasminogen activation axis in radical prostatectomy patients. Eur Urol 2009;55(5):1124–33.

33. Boyd LK, Mao X, Lu YJ. The complexity of prostate cancer: genomic alterations and heterogeneity. Nat Rev Urol 2012;9(11):652–64.

34. Shah RB, Bentley J, Jeffery Z, et al. Heterogeneity of PTEN and ERG expression in prostate cancer on core needle biopsies: implications for cancer risk stratification and biomarker sampling. Hum Pathol 2015;46(5):698–706.

35. Burger M, Catto JW, Dalbagni G, et al. Epidemiology and risk factors of urothelial bladder cancer. Eur Urol 2013;63(2):234–41.

36. Casella R, Shariat SF, Monoski MA, et al. Urinary levels of urokinase-type plasminogen activator and its receptor in the detection of bladder carcinoma. Cancer 2002;95(12):2494–9.

37. Bhuvarahamurthy V, Schroeder J, Denkert C, et al. In situ gene expression of urokinase-type plasminogen activator and its receptor in transitional cell carcinoma of the human bladder. Oncol Rep 2004; 12(4):909–13.

38. El-Kott AF, Khalil AM, El-Kenawy Ael M. Immunohistochemical expressions of uPA and its receptor uPAR and their prognostic significant in urinary bladder carcinoma. Int Urol Nephrol 2004;36(3): 417–23.

39. Seddighzadeh M, Steineck G, Larsson P, et al. Expression of UPA and UPAR is associated with the clinical course of urinary bladder neoplasms. Int J Cancer 2002;99(5):721–6.

40. Dohn LH, Illemann M, Hoyer-Hansen G, et al. Urokinase-type plasminogen activator receptor (uPAR) expression is associated with T-stage and survival in urothelial carcinoma of the bladder. Urol Oncol 2015;33(4):165.e15–24.

41. Dohn LH, Pappot H, Iversen BR, et al. uPAR expression pattern in patients with urothelial carcinoma of the bladder–possible clinical implications. PLoS One 2015;10(8):e0135824.

42. Shariat SF, Monoski MA, Andrews B, et al. Association of plasma urokinase-type plasminogen activator and its receptor with clinical outcome in patients undergoing radical cystectomy for transitional cell carcinoma of the bladder. Urology 2003;61(5): 1053–8.

43. Salajegheh M, Rudnicke A, Smith TJ. Expression of urokinase-type plasminogen activator receptor (uPAR) in primary central nervous system neoplasms. Appl Immunohistochem Mol Morphol 2005;13:184–9.

44. Mohanam S, Gladson CL, Rao CN, et al. Biological significance of the expression of urokinase-type plasminogen activator receptors (uPARs) in brain tumors. Front Biosci 1999;4:D178–87.

45. Yamamoto M, Sawaya R, Mohanam S, et al. Expression and localization of urokinase-type plasminogen activator receptor in human gliomas. Cancer Res 1994;54(18):5016–20.

46. Hirata K, Tamaki N. uPAR as a glioma imaging target. J Nucl Med 2016;57(2):169–70.

47. Wykosky J, Hu J, Gomez GG, et al. A urokinase receptor-Bim signaling axis emerges during EGFR inhibitor resistance in mutant EGFR glioblastoma. Cancer Res 2015;75(2):394–404.

48. Torre LA, Siegel RL, Ward EM, et al. Global cancer incidence and mortality rates and trends–an update. Cancer Epidemiol Biomarkers Prev 2016;25(1):16–27.

49. Cantero D, Friess H, Deflorin J, et al. Enhanced expression of urokinase plasminogen activator and its receptor in pancreatic carcinoma. Br J Cancer 1997;75(3):388–95.

50. Harvey SR, Hurd TC, Markus G, et al. Evaluation of urinary plasminogen activator, its receptor, matrix metalloproteinase-9, and von Willebrand factor in pancreatic cancer. Clin Cancer Res 2003;9(13):4935–43.

51. Gorantla B, Asuthkar S, Rao JS, et al. Suppression of the uPAR-uPA system retards angiogenesis, invasion, and in vivo tumor development in pancreatic cancer cells. Mol Cancer Res 2011;9(4):377–89.

52. Hildenbrand R, Niedergethmann M, Marx A, et al. Amplification of the urokinase-type plasminogen activator receptor (uPAR) gene in ductal pancreatic carcinomas identifies a clinically high-risk group. Am J Pathol 2009;174(6):2246–53.

53. Sorio C, Mafficini A, Furlan F, et al. Elevated urinary levels of urokinase-type plasminogen activator receptor (uPAR) in pancreatic ductal adenocarcinoma identify a clinically high-risk group. BMC cancer 2011;11:448.

54. Ploug M, Ostergaard S, Gardsvoll H, et al. Peptide-derived antagonists of the urokinase receptor. Affinity maturation by combinatorial chemistry, identification of functional epitopes, and inhibitory effect on cancer cell intravasation. Biochemistry 2001;40(40):12157–68.

55. Persson M, Madsen J, Ostergaard S, et al. Quantitative PET of human urokinase-type plasminogen activator receptor with 64Cu-DOTA-AE105: implications for visualizing cancer invasion. J Nucl Med 2012;53(1):138–45.

56. Li ZB, Niu G, Wang H, et al. Imaging of urokinase-type plasminogen activator receptor expression using a 64Cu-labeled linear peptide antagonist by microPET. Clin Cancer Res 2008;14(15):4758–66.

57. Persson M, Hosseini M, Madsen J, et al. Improved PET imaging of uPAR expression using new (64) Cu-labeled cross-bridged peptide ligands: comparative in vitro and in vivo studies. Theranostics 2013;3(9):618–32.

58. Persson M, Liu H, Madsen J, et al. First (18)F-labeled ligand for PET imaging of uPAR: in vivo studies in human prostate cancer xenografts. Nucl Med Biol 2013;40(5):618–24.

59. Persson M, Madsen J, Ostergaard S, et al. (68)Ga-labeling and in vivo evaluation of a uPAR binding DOTA- and NODAGA-conjugated peptide for PET imaging of invasive cancers. Nucl Med Biol 2012;39(4):560–9.

60. Persson M, Nedergaard MK, Brandt-Larsen M, et al. Urokinase-type plasminogen activator receptor as a potential PET biomarker in glioblastoma. J Nucl Med 2016;57(2):272–8.

61. Lin L, Gardsvoll H, Huai Q, et al. Structure-based engineering of species selectivity in the interaction between urokinase and its receptor: implication for preclinical cancer therapy. J Biol Chem 2010;285(14):10982–92.

62. Deloar HM, Fujiwara T, Shidahara M, et al. Estimation of absorbed dose for 2-[F-18]fluoro-2-deoxy-D-glucose using whole-body positron emission tomography and magnetic resonance imaging. Eur J Nucl Med 1998;25(6):565–74.

63. Leiblich A, Stevens D, Sooriakumaran P. The utility of molecular imaging in prostate cancer. Curr Urol Rep 2016;17(3):26.

64. Weissleder R, Schwaiger MC, Gambhir SS, et al. Imaging approaches to optimize molecular therapies. Sci Transl Med 2016;8(355):355ps316.

65. Mazar AP, Ahn RW, O'Halloran TV. Development of novel therapeutics targeting the urokinase plasminogen activator receptor (uPAR) and their translation toward the clinic. Curr Pharm Des 2011;17(19):1970–8.

66. Rabbani SA, Ateeq B, Arakelian A, et al. An anti-urokinase plasminogen activator receptor antibody (ATN-658) blocks prostate cancer invasion, migration, growth, and experimental skeletal metastasis in vitro and in vivo. Neoplasia 2010;12(10):778–88.

67. Persson M, Juhl K, Rasmussen P, et al. uPAR targeted radionuclide therapy with (177)Lu-DOTA-AE105 inhibits dissemination of metastatic prostate cancer. Mol Pharm 2014;11(8):2796–806.

68. Brabander T, Teunissen JJ, Van Eijck CH, et al. Peptide receptor radionuclide therapy of neuroendocrine tumours. Best Pract Res Clin Endocrinol Metab 2016;30(1):103–14.

69. Persson M, Rasmussen P, Madsen J, et al. New peptide receptor radionuclide therapy of invasive cancer cells: in vivo studies using 177Lu-DOTA-AE105 targeting uPAR in human colorectal cancer xenografts. Nucl Med Biol 2012;39(7):962–9.

Magnetic Resonance-based Motion Correction for Quantitative PET in Simultaneous PET-MR Imaging

Yothin Rakvongthai, PhD[a], Georges El Fakhri, PhD[b],*

KEYWORDS

• PET-MR • Respiratory motion • Cardiac motion • MR-based motion correction

KEY POINTS

- Simultaneous PET-MR offers a tool that can be used for correcting the motion in PET images by using high-quality anatomic information from MR imaging.
- The MR-based PET motion correction consists of 2 parts: estimating deformation field or motion field from MR data, and creating motion-free PET images using the estimated deformation field.
- Several phantom animal and patient studies have validated that MR-based motion correction strategies have great promise for quantitative PET imaging in simultaneous PET-MR.

INTRODUCTION

Patient motion degrades image quality and quantitation of PET images, and is an obstacle to quantitative PET imaging. The blurring owing to motion leads to the underestimation of tracer uptake values,[1,2] and the reduction of lesion detectability,[3–6] especially for small lesions. For whole-body PET scanners, the intrinsic spatial resolution is approximately 4 mm,[7,8] which could not be achieved in clinical thoracic and abdomen studies due to unavoidable patient motion. In particular, during respiration, the diaphragm and the liver move up to 28 mm and 17 mm,[9] respectively, which severely affects detection of lesions in the liver dome.[3,4] Moreover, the heart moves up to 9 mm during free breathing.[9] In addition to blurring, the motion creates discrepancy between the emission and attenuation data, which leads to confounding artifacts in PET images, and thus reducing PET quantitative accuracy.

There are several ways to generate PET images in the presence of motion. First, one can mistakenly ignore the motion by assuming that the object to be imaged has no motion, and reconstruct the PET image (this is called the no motion correction or the uncorrection method). There have been research studies that attempt to overcome the effects of motion. Tracking systems using external devices[10] that link external movements to internal organs' trajectories has been proposed, but the errors are still substantial. PET data alone also can be used to estimate the motion; however, its accuracy is limited by the relatively low spatial resolution of PET, and it only works well for regions with high activity.[11] Another widely used scheme to deal with motion is the gating method, which freezes the cardiac and/or the respiratory motions. In this case, the motion trajectory is subdivided into phases and acquired PET data are binned into multiple frames or gates according a specific motion phase. Consequently, the PET image is reconstructed from one chosen reference

The authors have nothing to disclose.
[a] Division of Nuclear Medicine, Department of Radiology, Faculty of Medicine, Chulalongkorn University, Bangkok 10330, Thailand; [b] Gordon Center for Medical Imaging, Department of Radiology, Massachusetts General Hospital, Harvard Medical School, Boston, MA 02114, USA
* Corresponding author.
E-mail address: elfakhri@pet.mgh.harvard.edu

PET Clin 12 (2017) 321–327
http://dx.doi.org/10.1016/j.cpet.2017.02.004
1556-8598/17/© 2017 Elsevier Inc. All rights reserved.

frame to represent a motion-free PET image. Nevertheless, this strategy uses only a small fraction of the emission data for reconstructing the PET image in each individual gate. This leads to a tradeoff of the image's signal-to-noise-ratio (SNR) and the total scan time, and, therefore, it is not optimal.

Simultaneous PET-magnetic resonance imaging (MR imaging) offers a tool that can be used for correcting the motion in PET images by using high-quality anatomic information from MR imaging. Unlike in PET-computed tomography (CT), motion-induced blurring can be alleviated in PET-MR without additional radiation exposure or loss of SNR while both emission data and data used for creating motion fields are acquired concurrently. The combination between PET and MR also allows us to take advantage of both modalities.

The MR-based PET motion correction consists of 2 parts: estimating deformation field or motion field from MR data, and creating motion-free PET images using the estimated deformation field. This so-called motion field or deformation field is a vector field representing the displacement of all individual voxels from every motion phase to a chosen reference phase. To perform motion estimation from MR imaging, the motion fields are extracted from measured MR data that are acquired under MR imaging acquisition protocols especially designed for fast dynamic imaging. In addition to PET motion correction, motion estimation also is used to generate the time-dependent attenuation maps to be used for PET image reconstruction. To create the motion-corrected PET image, the first approach uses data from all gates by reconstructing PET images of all frames, and transforming them into the reference frame. The transformed images that result are averaged to have the motion-corrected PET image. Instead of transforming PET images in the postreconstruction step, another approach incorporates the transformation into the reconstruction system model, and obtains the motion-corrected PET image in a single reconstruction framework.

MAGNETIC RESONANCE-BASED MOTION MEASUREMENT AND MOTION FIELD ESTIMATION

Two major causes of motion-induced blurring artifacts are the respiratory motion and the cardiac motion. This section discusses how to measure the respiratory and the cardiac motions using MR imaging to assist PET motion correction in thoracic/abdomen and cardiac PET-MR imaging.[12,13]

A dedicated MR imaging pulse sequence called NAV-TrueFISP was developed to measure the respiratory motion for lower abdomen PET-MR imaging.[14] It takes advantage of specific contrast of single-slice steady-state free precession MR imaging acquisitions (TrueFISP) to produce anatomic landmarks in homogeneous tissues in the lower abdomen, such as liver, by combining TrueFISP with interleaving pencil-beam navigator echoes. Collected before each TrueFISP acquisition, these navigators track the lung-liver interface during the respiratory cycle. The resulted internal motion surrogates yield accurate binning of simultaneously acquired PET-MR data into respiratory phase, which is performed based on the navigator amplitude. As a result, gated MR image volumes can be used for computing the respiratory motion field. Another approach used a navigator-encapsulated golden angle radial fast low-angle shot (FLASH) pulse sequence to obtain time-dependent lung MR images in pulmonary PET-MR imaging.[15]

It should be mentioned that a patient study in abdominal, thoracic, and cardiac imaging compared performance of several methods to acquire motion field in simultaneous PET-MR.[16]

For correcting motion in cardiac imaging, MR-based cardiac motion estimation involves 2 motion types: cardiac motion and respiratory motion. The motion field for these 2 types are measured separately, and are combined to create the motion field between any cardiac or respiratory phase to the reference phase.

The cardiac motion can be traced using the tagged MR imaging technique, in which series of parallel strips are created on the muscle tissue. These strips are called tags, which are induced by periodic magnetization modulation due to specific radiofrequency (RF)/gradients series. A series of MR images is obtained in which the tags are visible and their deformation is used to estimate cardiac motion. The sequence is also navigated by a pencil-beam navigator, allowing the acquisition of tagged MR data only at end-expiration respiratory phase. Electrocardiogram signals and navigators are acquired simultaneously for labeling each PET coincidence into a cardiac and respiratory phase. To speed up from regular tagging acquisition (10 minutes), an accelerated acquisition has been developed using advanced MR techniques, such as compressed sensing.[17] It should be noted that although the tagged MR imaging technique has been successfully used in phantoms and abdominal imaging of rabbits and nonhuman primates, it is impractical for respiratory motion estimation in human studies because tag lines fade rapidly to capture the longer human breathing cycle.[14,15]

Deformation fields from MR imaging is essential for PET motion correction. Accurate motion correction needs volumetric motion fields obtained from nonrigid registration of anatomic images acquired simultaneously with PET. To estimate the motion field from a series of MR image volumes, B-spline nonrigid image registration, which is based on the sum of squared difference (SSD) or mutual information (MI),[18] can be used. Denote an MR image volume at a given motion phase k by $f(k,\mathbf{v})$. Given that the SSD is used, the motion fields are the solution to this minimization problem[14]:

$$\hat{g}(k \to k', \mathbf{v}) = argmin_g \left[\frac{1}{N} \sum_{\mathbf{v}} \left(f(k, g(k \to k', \mathbf{v})) \right. \right.$$
$$\left. \left. - f(k', \mathbf{v})^2 \right) + \beta R(g(k \to k', \mathbf{v})) \right],$$

where $\mathbf{v}$ is the voxel position, N is the total number of voxels, β is a regularization parameter, and $R(\cdot)$ is a regularizer. The regularization is present to achieve stable and realistic solution because motion estimation is an ill-posed inverse problem.

MOTION CORRECTION IN PET RECONSTRUCTION

The motion-corrected PET image, which is the PET image corresponding to a given reference frame or gate, can be obtained by using 2 approaches: the reconstruct-transform-average (RTA)[19–21] and the motion-compensated image reconstruction (MCIR)[22–26] methods. In the first approach, the PET image in each frame is reconstructed separately, and is then transformed back into the reference frame. All resulting transformed images are averaged to generate the motion-corrected PET image. Unlike the RTA method, the MCIR method includes the transformation in the PET system model, and reconstructs the motion-corrected PET image in a single reconstruction framework. This section discusses these 2 PET motion correction approaches.

Reconstruct-Transform-Average Approach

Once the deformation fields mapping the PET image in the reference frame to all frames are obtained, the motion-corrected PET image in the reference frame can be reconstructed by using the RTA method. To begin with, the PET system model for frame k is given by

$$\bar{y}_k = H_k x_k + s_k + r_k,$$

where $\bar{y}_k$ is the mean PET sinogram in frame k, $\mathbf{x}_k$ is the PET image, and $\mathbf{s}_k$ and $\mathbf{r}_k$ are the average scattered and random counts in the same frame. The system matrix $\mathbf{H}_k$ for frame k incorporates the detector sensitivity, detector blurring, frame-dependent attenuation factors, forward-projection operator, and the warping operator transforming the reference frame to the kth frame. Mathematically, the system matrix can be written as

$$H_k = NBA_k G,$$

where $\mathbf{N}$ is a diagonal matrix accounting for the detector normalization factors, $\mathbf{B}$ models the detector blurring effects in the sinogram domain, $\mathbf{A}_k$ is a diagonal matrix representing the attenuation correction factors for each frame, $\mathbf{G}$ is the forward-projection operator whose (i,j)-th element represents the probability that an emission in voxel j is detected in detector bin i. A standard reconstruction method, such as the ordered-subset expectation maximization (OSEM) algorithm, can be used to obtain the estimated PET image in frame k, $\hat{x}_k$. The final motion-corrected PET image in the RTA method is then given by

$$\hat{x}_{RTA} = \frac{1}{K} \sum_k M_k^{-1} \hat{x}_k,$$

where $\mathbf{M}_k$ is an interpolation matrix accounting for warping operator for transformation from the reference frame to the kth frame, and K is the total number of motion frames. Another variant of this RTA method has been proposed[27] in which each frame in the average step is weighted by the reciprocal of the relative amplitude change in that frame.

Motion-Compensated Image Reconstruction Approach

Even though there are studies[27,28] showing that motion correction with the RTA method yields improvement in terms of image quality in comparison with the uncorrected method, the RTA method involves the transformation in the postreconstruction step, and therefore is suboptimal. A more sophisticated method for applying motion correction in PET modifies the image reconstruction process. This method is referred to as MCIR. Unlike the RTA method, in which the transformation is performed after reconstruction, the MCIR method incorporates the transformation in the system model, and reconstructs the motion-corrected PET image in the reference frame in a single reconstruction framework.[14,15,25,29–32]

In this case, the PET system model can be written as

$$\bar{y}_k = P_k x + s_k + r_k \, ,$$

where x is the PET image in the reference frame to be reconstructed. In addition to all physical effects, the system matrix P_k for frame k in MCIR also incorporates the warping operator transforming the reference frame to the kth frame. The system matrix in MCIR can be written as

$$P_k = NBA_k GM_k \, .$$

To reconstruct the motion-corrected image in the MCIR framework, the widely used OSEM algorithm can also be extended, and its update equation at iteration i is given by[14]

$$x^{[i+1]} = \frac{x^{[i]}}{\sum_k w_k M_k^T G^T A_k BN1}$$
$$\times \sum_k M_k^T G^T B \frac{y_k}{BGM_k x^{[i]} + (A_k N)^{-1}(s+r)} \, ,$$

where 1 is a column vector whose elements are all 1, y_k is the measured PET sinogram in frame k, and w_k is the relative duration of frame k. It is assumed that the effects of random and scatter coincidences do not change with the motion frames;

therefore, the subscripts of s and r are omitted. This iterative approach yields the motion-corrected PET image in the MCIR framework, $\hat{x}_{MCIR}$. It should be noted that in addition to the OSEM, the maximum a posteriori (MAP)[33,34] reconstruction also can be used for the MCIR framework. A MAP reconstruction with quadratic penalty function as a prior together with a preconditioned conjugate gradient algorithm was proposed for motion correction in lung PET imaging with integrated PET-MR.[15] **Fig. 1** illustrates the diagram for the RTA and the MCIR methods for PET motion correction. Several phantom and patient studies[35–38] compared both approaches based on the OSEM image reconstruction and regularized reconstruction, and reported that the MCIR approach yielded better motion-corrected images as compared with the RTA approach.

IMPACT OF MOTION CORRECTION ON QUANTITATIVE PET USING PET-MAGNETIC RESONANCE

Applying MR-based motion correction in simultaneous PET-MR yields improved quantitative PET imaging. This section presents the results of motion correction and its impact on quantitative PET using simultaneous PET-MR.

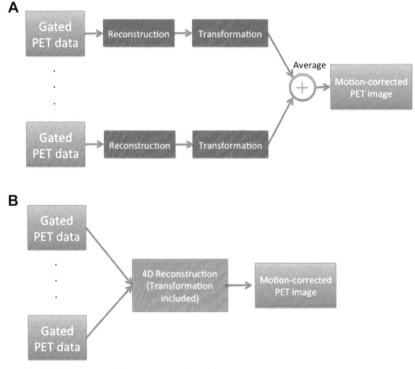

Fig. 1. Diagram for (A) the RTA and (B) MCIR methods for PET motion correction.

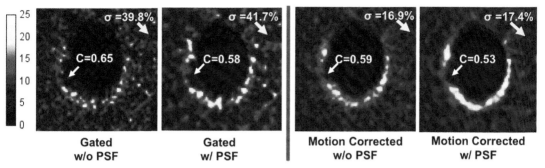

Fig. 2. Slices of PET images from a moving cardiac phantom study comparing the images without motion correction and the motion-corrected images (without and with PSF modeling). (*Adapted from* Petibon Y, Ouyang J, Zhu X, et al. Cardiac motion compensation and resolution modeling in simultaneous PET-MR: a cardiac lesion detection study. Phys Med Biol 2013;58(7):2098; with permission.)

Cardiac imaging is one of several areas that benefits from advancement of PET motion correction in simultaneous PET/MR.[14,32] It was reported[32] that MR-based motion correction yielded an improvement in contrast recovery of 34% to 206% in comparison with the no motion correction method, and in myocardial defect detectability of 115% to 136% and 62% to 235% as compared with the gating and no motion correction methods, respectively. In a plaque imaging study,[9] motion correction improved plaque detectability in terms of the channelized Hotelling observer–SNR by 105% to 128% and plaque contrast by 30% to 71% as compared with no motion correction, and by 348% and 396% as compared with the gating and dual (cardiac-respiratory) gating methods. Fig. 2 shows impact of motion correction in cardiac lesion detection. Motion correction visually and quantitatively had better noise control while maintaining comparable contrast as compared with the gating method.

Motion correction also has impact on oncologic PET imaging. A quantitative oncologic PET-MR imaging framework involving MR-based motion correction and point spread function (PSF) compensation has been proposed.[14] The study therein showed the improvement due to motion correction in tumor delineation (see also Fig. 3), and also suggested that the gain of motion correction was more pronounced when PSF modeling is incorporated and vice versa. There have been studies in several oncologic applications that reported[15,38,39] that the respiratory compensation improved PET quantitative accuracy as compared with the no motion correction method in several aspects including contrast-to-noise ratio (CNR) (increased by 19%–190%), the peak standardized uptake value (SUV) and maximum SUV (increased on average by 23.1% and 34.5%), the lesion size (reduced by 60.4% on average), and the lesion position (change of 60.9%). In comparison with the gating method, the motion correction method show improvement on the CNR by 6% to 51%.[15]

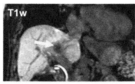

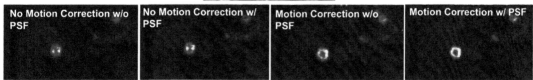

Fig. 3. Slices of PET images from a patient study comparing the images without motion correction and the motion-corrected images (without and with PSF modeling). Notice the heterogeneity of uptake in the lesion (indicated by the *arrow* in the T1-weighted MR image) revealed in motioned corrected images. (*Adapted from* Petibon Y, Huang C, Ouyang J, et al. Relative role of motion and PSF compensation in whole-body oncologic PET-MR imaging. Med Phys 2014; 41:042503; with permission.)

SUMMARY

Motion degrades image quality and quantitation of PET images, and is an obstacle to quantitative PET imaging. Simultaneous PET-MR offers a tool that can be used for correcting the motion in PET images by using anatomic information from MR imaging acquired concurrently. Motion correction can be performed by transforming a set of reconstructed PET images into the same frame or by incorporating the transformation into the system model and reconstructing the motion-corrected image. Several phantom and patient studies in cardiac and oncologic phantoms demonstrated the significant improvement of PET quantitative accuracy such as CNR, SUV, and lesion detectability by motion correction as compared with the gating or the no motion correction methods. Therefore, MR-based motion correction has shown great promise to make quantitative PET imaging on simultaneous PET-MR possible.

ACKNOWLEDGMENTS

The authors thank Dr Yoann Petibon for his contribution to results presented in this article.

REFERENCES

1. Liu C, Pierce LA 2nd, Alessio AM, et al. The impact of respiratory motion on tumor quantification and delineation in static PET/CT imaging. Phys Med Biol 2009;54(24):7345–62.
2. Nehmeh SA, Erdi YE, Pan T, et al. Four-dimensional (4D) PET/CT imaging of the thorax. Med Phys 2004; 31(12):3179–86.
3. Papathanassiou D, Becker S, Amir R, et al. Respiratory motion artefact in the liver dome on FDG PET/CT: comparison of attenuation correction with CT and a caesium external source. Eur J Nucl Med Mol Imaging 2005;32(12):1422–8.
4. Sureshbabu W, Mawlawi O. PET/CT imaging artifacts. J Nucl Med Technol 2005;33(3):156–61.
5. Nehmeh SA, Erdi YE, Ling CC, et al. Effect of respiratory gating on quantifying PET images of lung cancer. J Nucl Med 2002;43(7):876–81.
6. Polycarpou I, Tsoumpas C, King AP, et al. Impact of respiratory motion correction and spatial resolution on lesion detection in PET: a simulation study based on real MR dynamic data. Phys Med Biol 2014;59(3): 697–713.
7. Stickel JR, Cherry SR. High-resolution PET detector design: modelling components of intrinsic spatial resolution. Phys Med Biol 2005;50(2):179–95.
8. Wiant D, Gersh JA, Bennett M, et al. Evaluation of the spatial dependence of the point spread function in 2D PET image reconstruction using LOR-OSEM. Med Phys 2010;37(3):1169–82.
9. Boucher L, Rodrigue S, Lecomte R, et al. Respiratory gating for 3-dimensional PET of the thorax: feasibility and initial results. J Nucl Med 2004; 45(2):214–9.
10. Rahmim A, Rousset O, Zaidi H. Strategies for motion tracking and correction in PET. PET Clin 2007;2(2): 251–66.
11. Vandenberghe S, Marsden PK. PET-MRI: a review of challenges and solutions in the development of integrated multimodality imaging. Phys Med Biol 2015;60(4):R115–54.
12. Ouyang J, Li Q, El Fakhri G. Magnetic resonance-based motion correction for positron emission tomography imaging. Semin Nucl Med 2013;43(1): 60–7.
13. Ouyang J, Petibon Y, Huang C, et al. Quantitative simultaneous positron emission tomography and magnetic resonance imaging. J Med Imaging (Bellingham) 2014;1(3):033502.
14. Petibon Y, Huang C, Ouyang J, et al. Relative role of motion and PSF compensation in whole-body oncologic PET-MR imaging. Med Phys 2014;41(4): 042503.
15. Dutta J, Huang C, Li Q, et al. Pulmonary imaging using respiratory motion compensated simultaneous PET/MR. Med Phys 2015;42(7):4227–40.
16. Furst S, Grimm R, Hong I, et al. Motion correction strategies for integrated PET/MR. J Nucl Med 2015;56(2):261–9.
17. Huang C, Petibon Y, Ouyang J, et al. Accelerated acquisition of tagged MRI for cardiac motion correction in simultaneous PET-MR: phantom and patient studies. Med Phys 2015;42(2):1087–97.
18. Chun SY, Fessler JA. A simple regularizer for B-spline nonrigid image registration that encourages local invertibility. IEEE J Sel Top Signal Process 2009;3(1):159–69.
19. Picard Y, Thompson CJ. Motion correction of PET images using multiple acquisition frames. IEEE Trans Med Imaging 1997;16(2):137–44.
20. Klein G, Reutter B, Huesman R. Non-rigid summing of gated PET via optical flow. IEEE Trans Nucl Sci 1997;44(4):1509–12.
21. Dawood M, Lang N, Jiang X, et al. Lung motion correction on respiratory gated 3-D PET/CT images. IEEE Trans Med Imaging 2006;25(4):476–85.
22. Qiao F, Pan T, Clark JW Jr, et al. A motion-incorporated reconstruction method for gated PET studies. Phys Med Biol 2006;51(15):3769–83.
23. Li T, Thorndyke B, Schreibmann E, et al. Model-based image reconstruction for four-dimensional PET. Med Phys 2006;33(5):1288–98.
24. Lamare F, Ledesma Carbayo MJ, Cresson T, et al. List-mode-based reconstruction for respiratory motion correction in PET using non-rigid body transformations. Phys Med Biol 2007;52(17): 5187–204.

25. Petibon Y, El Fakhri G, Nezafat R, et al. Towards coronary plaque imaging using simultaneous PET-MR: a simulation study. Phys Med Biol 2014;59(5):1203–22.

26. Rahmim A, Bloomfield P, Houle S, et al. Motion compensation in histogram-mode and list-mode em reconstructions: beyond the event-driven approach. IEEE Trans Nucl Sci 2004;51(5):2588–96.

27. Wurslin C, Schmidt H, Martirosian P, et al. Respiratory motion correction in oncologic PET using T1-weighted MR imaging on a simultaneous whole-body PET/MR system. J Nucl Med 2013; 54(3):464–71.

28. Grimm R, Furst S, Souvatzoglou M, et al. Self-gated MRI motion modeling for respiratory motion compensation in integrated PET/MRI. Med Image Anal 2015;19(1):110–20.

29. Guerin B, Cho S, Chun SY, et al. Nonrigid PET motion compensation in the lower abdomen using simultaneous tagged-MRI and PET imaging. Med Phys 2011;38(6):3025–38.

30. Chun SY, Reese TG, Ouyang J, et al. MRI-based nonrigid motion correction in simultaneous PET/MRI. J Nucl Med 2012;53(8):1284–91.

31. Huang C, Ackerman JL, Petibon Y, et al. Motion compensation for brain PET imaging using wireless MR active markers in simultaneous PET-MR: phantom and non-human primate studies. Neuroimage 2014;91:129–37.

32. Petibon Y, Ouyang J, Zhu X, et al. Cardiac motion compensation and resolution modeling in simultaneous PET-MR: a cardiac lesion detection study. Phys Med Biol 2013;58(7):2085–102.

33. Qi J, Leahy RM. A theoretical study of the contrast recovery and variance of MAP reconstructions from PET data. IEEE Trans Med Imaging 1999; 18(4):293–305.

34. Leahy RM, Qi J. Statistical approaches in quantitative positron emission tomography. Statistics and Computing 2000;10(2):147–65.

35. Dikaios N, Izquierdo-Garcia D, Graves MJ, et al. MRI-based motion correction of thoracic PET: initial comparison of acquisition protocols and correction strategies suitable for simultaneous PET/MRI systems. Eur Radiol 2012;22(2):439–46.

36. Polycarpou I, Tsoumpas C, Marsden PK. Analysis and comparison of two methods for motion correction in PET imaging. Med Phys 2012;39(10):6474–83.

37. Tsoumpas C, Polycarpou I, Thielemans K, et al. The effect of regularization in motion compensated PET image reconstruction: a realistic numerical 4D simulation study. Phys Med Biol 2013;58(6):1759–73.

38. Fayad H, Schmidt H, Wuerslin C, et al. Reconstruction-incorporated respiratory motion correction in clinical simultaneous PET/MR imaging for oncology applications. J Nucl Med 2015;56(6):884–9.

39. Manber R, Thielemans K, Hutton BF, et al. Practical PET respiratory motion correction in clinical PET/MR. J Nucl Med 2015;56(6):890–6.

PET Imaging for Early Detection of Alzheimer's Disease

From Pathologic to Physiologic Biomarkers

Weiqi Bao, MD, PhD[a], Hongmei Jia, PhD[b],
Sjoerd Finnema, PhD[c], Zhengxin Cai, PhD[c],
Richard E. Carson, PhD[c], Yiyun Henry Huang, PhD[c],*

KEYWORDS

- Alzheimer's disease • PET imaging • Synaptic density • Beta-amyloid • Tau protein • Cholinergic
- Inflammation • SV2A

KEY POINTS

- PET imaging biomarkers are important for Alzheimer's disease research and diagnosis.
- PET imaging of β-amyloid protein plaques has contributed greatly to the understanding of Alzheimer's disease and its progression, and development of therapeutic agents for its treatment.
- PET imaging of other biomarkers for Alzheimer's disease will help unravel its etiology and topographic progression.
- Measurement of synaptic density through PET imaging of the synaptic vesicle glycoprotein 2A (SV2A) may provide a tool for early diagnosis of Alzheimer's disease.

INTRODUCTION

Alzheimer's disease (AD) affects more than 35 million people worldwide, and the number is estimated to quadruple in 40 years if there remains no cure.[1–4] AD is characterized by the presence of pathologic lesions in brain, mainly β-amyloid (Aβ) plaques and neurofibrillary tangles, as well as hyperphosphorylated tau protein aggregates, with significant loss of neurons and atrophy at later stages, and can be definitively diagnosed only with postmortem histology staining of brain tissues. Early symptoms of AD are marked by the impairment of declarative memories, and accumulating evidence suggests that this occurs as the hippocampal synapses are compromised by soluble Aβ protein oligomers during the earliest phase of AD.[5–7] Evidence also suggests that neuropathological development occurs over many years, if not decades, before any presentation of clinical symptoms, with mild cognitive impairment (MCI) being a prodrome of AD, and synapse loss occurring before the accumulation of Aβ.[8]

From a diagnostic perspective, AD is increasingly viewed along a continuum from preclinical AD, to MCI, and to AD dementia.[4] PET imaging is increasingly used in AD diagnosis to measure physiologic biomarkers (eg, glucose metabolism with ^{18}F-fluorodeoxyglucose [^{18}F-FDG]), and pathologic biomarkers such as Aβ.[9] In addition, imaging of other physiologic biomarkers targeted at the cholinergic system and pathologic biomarkers

Disclosure Statement: The authors have nothing to disclose.
[a] PET Center, Huanshan Hospital, Fudan University, No. 518, East Wuzhong Road, Xuhui District, Shanghai 200235, China; [b] Key Laboratory of Radiopharmaceuticals, Ministry of Education, College of Chemistry, Beijing Normal University, No. 19, Xinjiekouwai Street, Beijing 10075, China; [c] Department of Radiology and Biomedical Imaging, PET Center, Yale University School of Medicine, PO Box 208048, New Haven, CT 06520-8048, USA
* Corresponding author.
E-mail address: henry.huang@yale.edu

such as tau protein aggregates and AD-associated neuroinflammation have also been explored for diagnosis and progression monitoring of AD. A more recent development is the emergence of PET radioligands for direct measurement of synaptic density for use in AD imaging. In this article, we review the application of PET biomarkers available for AD imaging, and provide comments on the prospects of these imaging biomarkers for the early diagnosis of AD, monitoring of disease progression, and assessment of treatment effects.

PET IMAGING OF PATHOLOGIC BIOMARKERS IN ALZHEIMER'S DISEASE
Radiotracers for β-Amyloids

The amyloid cascade hypothesis points to formation of Aβ plaques and neurofibrillary tangles as the central event in the pathogenesis of AD.[10,11] Aβ is generated by the sequential cleavage of amyloid precursor protein (APP) by β-secretase and the γ-secretase complex. β-secretase cleaves APP into soluble sAPPβ and the remaining C-terminal fragment. The latter is then cleaved by γ-secretase into Aβ$_{42}$ and the Aβ intracellular cytoplasmic domain. Aβ aggregation, including different stages of aggregates from soluble oligomers to insoluble fibrils in plaques, impairs synaptic function and ultimately damages neurons, leading to cell death, cognitive impairment, and finally dementia.[12] The target of in vivo amyloid imaging agents is Aβ deposition, in all forms of Aβ plaques as well as cerebral amyloid angiopathy.

Five Aβ-specific radioligands have been developed for PET imaging of patients with AD (**Fig. 1**).[13,14] Among these, ^{11}C-Pittsburgh compound-B (^{11}C-PIB) was the first used in patients with AD and remains the "gold standard" amyloid PET agent. Three ^{18}F-labeled Aβ agents, ^{18}F-florbetapir (AV-45, Amyvid), ^{18}F-flutemetamol

(GE-067, Vizamyl), and ^{18}F-florbetaben (AV-1, BAY94-9172, NeuraCeq), have been approved by the Food and Drug Administration (FDA) for clinical detection of Aβ in patients with AD. ^{18}F-NAV4694 (^{18}F-AZD4694) is a third-generation Aβ probe with similar imaging characteristics to ^{11}C-PIB.[15,16]

[11]C-Pittsburgh compound-B
[11]C-PIB is a PET radioligand derived from the Aβ staining agent thioflavin-T. In the very first study of in vivo Aβ imaging in patients with AD, initiated in 2002 and published in 2004,[17] marked increase in ^{11}C-PIB uptake was observed in brain areas with high levels of amyloid plaques. Since then, numerous PET imaging studies with ^{11}C-PIB have been performed in patients with autosomal dominant AD, MCI, and cognitively healthy controls, and the results described in several review articles.[13,14,18,19] As confirmed by autopsy and immunohistochemical staining of brain slices, the regional retention of ^{11}C-PIB reflects the regional density of Aβ plaques with higher densities in the frontal cortex, cingulate gyrus, precuneus, striatum, parietal cortex, and lateral temporal cortex, and lower in the occipital cortex, sensorimotor cortex, and mesial temporal cortex.[19] A proportion of 10% to 30% of healthy elderly subjects have significant ^{11}C-PIB retention, which is strongly related to the presence of ApoE4 genotype, and associated with a greater risk of cognitive decline and a faster rate of brain atrophy. Approximately 60% to 75% of subjects with MCI were found to have AD-like ^{11}C-PIB retention. Longitudinal studies have indicated that Aβ accumulation is a slow process that lasts over 20 to 30 years, that healthy elderly subjects and subjects with MCI with increased ^{11}C-PIB retention present faster rates of Aβ deposition, which was significantly associated with faster memory decline and disease progression, and that subjects with MCI

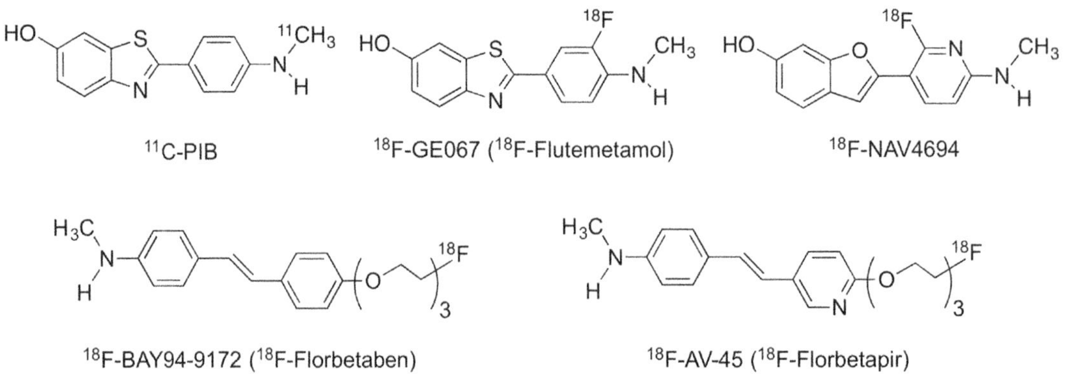

Fig. 1. Chemical structures of radiotracers for Aβ.

with high ^{11}C-PIB binding exhibit much more frequent conversion to AD than those with low ^{11}C-PIB binding.[20–24] However, it was also found that the degree of ^{11}C-PIB retention appears to display high intragroup variability among healthy elderly subjects, subjects with MCI, and patients with AD, and did not correlate with the severity of dementia in patients with AD, although elevated cortical retention of ^{11}C-PIB was observed. Therefore, ^{11}C-PIB PET is likely to have a prognostic role in the clinical evaluation of MCI by identifying subjects who have underlying AD pathophysiology and are therefore at high risk for further clinical decline.[25] In addition, ^{11}C-PIB PET imaging has also been used to screen cognitively healthy subjects into amyloid-positive and amyloid-negative subtypes for inclusion in clinical trials of anti-Aβ therapeutics, and to monitor the therapeutic outcomes.[26]

[18]F-florbetapir

Derived from the prototypical Aβ-staining agents Congo Red and Chrysamine G, ^{18}F-florbetapir was the first Aβ-specific PET radiotracer approved by the FDA in 2012. Later in 2013, marketing authorization for this radiotracer was also granted by the European Medicines Agency. In one study, a total of 229 patients participated in a clinical trial with ^{18}F-florbetapir. After receiving the results of the ^{18}F-florbetapir scan, diagnosis changed in 125 of 229, or 54.6% of cases, and diagnostic confidence increased by an average of 21.6%. A total of 199 of 229 or 86.9% of cases had at least 1 change in their management plan. Amyloid imaging results altered physician's diagnostic thinking, intended testing, and management of patients undergoing evaluation for cognitive decline.[27] In a recent follow-up study, it was reported that, of the 228 participants, diagnostic change occurred in 46 patients (79%) who had both a previous diagnosis of AD and an amyloid-negative scan, and in 16 (53%) of those with non-AD diagnosis and an amyloid-positive scan. Diagnostic confidence increased by 15.2% in amyloid-positive and decreased by 29.9% in amyloid-negative scans. These findings indicated that amyloid PET with ^{18}F-florbetapir, in addition to routine assessment in patients with cognitive impairment, has a significant effect on diagnosis, diagnostic confidence, and drug-treatment plan.[28]

[18]F-florbetaben

Similarly derived from the prototypical Aβ-staining agents Congo Red and Chrysamine G, ^{18}F-florbetaben was the first ^{18}F-labeled Aβ PET agent developed and approval has been granted in the United States, European Union, and South Korea

for its use in clinical PET imaging of Aβ in the brain of patients with AD. It was reported to have high diagnostic accuracy (as verified by postmortem histopathology) with good interreader agreement in detecting or excluding brain Aβ deposits in patients with various levels of cognitive function. Further, it appeared to require a short PET scan time of 15 to 20 minutes and to have high predictive values for reliably detecting or excluding amyloid pathology.[29] A recent report on early-phase acquisition of ^{18}F-florbetaben PET indicated that it also provided a metabolism-like image with good correlation to an ^{18}F-FDG PET scan, suggesting that early-phase acquisition with ^{18}F-florbetaben may serve as a surrogate marker for synaptic dysfunction.[30]

[18]F-flutemetamol

An analogue of ^{11}C-PIB and previously known as ^{18}F-GE067, ^{18}F-flutemetamol (3′-^{18}F-F-PIB) is also derived from the Aβ-staining agent thioflavin-T (see **Fig. 1**). A recent clinical trial of ^{18}F-flutemetamol PET imaging in 106 end-of-life subjects demonstrated a high specificity and sensitivity for Aβ pathology, and detection of a diagnostically relevant neuritic plaque burden.[31] It was reported that ^{18}F-flutemetamol PET imaging of the striatum in 68 subjects who later came to autopsy had reasonable accuracy for the detection of histologically demonstrated striatal Aβ plaques present at moderate or frequent densities (approximately 77%–83% sensitivity and 100% specificity), indicating that amyloid imaging of the cerebral cortex and striatum together may allow for a more accurate clinicopathological diagnosis of AD and for pathology-based clinical staging of AD.[32] Further, ^{18}F-flutemetamol PET changed clinical diagnosis, increased overall diagnostic confidence, and altered the patient management plan.[33]

^{18}F-NAV4694

^{18}F-NAV4694 (AZD4694) is a third-generation Aβ-specific imaging probe, and displays similar steric structure to ^{11}C-PIB (benzofuran and pyridinyl moieties vs benzothiazole and phenyl groups, respectively). It exhibited higher specific binding in the cortex and lower nonspecific binding in white matter than other ^{18}F-labeled Aβ radiotracers. Preliminary data indicated that ^{18}F-NAV4694 was able to differentiate AD from healthy controls. In addition, it showed a useful additive role for amyloid PET in atypical cases with an unclear diagnosis beyond the extensive workup of a tertiary memory clinic. Amyloid PET with ^{18}F-NAV4694 increased diagnostic confidence and led to clinically significant alterations

in management.[34] Recently, it was reported that ^{18}F-NAV4694 has slightly higher Aβ-specific binding and lower variance than ^{11}C-PIB, which are important properties for detecting early Aβ deposition and changes over time using the standard centiloid method.[35,36]

As detailed previously, several PET radiotracers for Aβ have been developed, and used increasingly in the clinic for AD diagnosis. These radiotracers have different binding and imaging characteristics, with all the ^{18}F-labeled radiotracers approved by the FDA having higher white matter binding than ^{11}C-PIB. A head-to-head comparison between ^{11}C-PIB and ^{18}F-labeled amyloid ligands has revealed significant overlap with respect to detection of amyloid plaques, linear regression slope, and diagnostic performance.[37,38] Quantitative comparison studies of PET data between ^{18}F-labeled radiotracers and ^{11}C-PIB acquired in the same subjects demonstrated high composite cortical binding correlation, indicating the translation of ^{11}C-PIB PET findings into the domain of ^{18}F-labeled radiotracers.[39,40] Further, significant correlation has been found between ^{11}C-PIB and ^{18}F-florbetapir across the different regions of interest examined in elderly healthy controls, amyloid-positive MCI, and AD groups in unrelated, matched patient populations. Discrimination between healthy controls and patients with AD was best for both tracers in the putamen.[37] On the other hand, ^{18}F-florbetapir was found to perform less well at discriminating between healthy controls and patients with AD than ^{11}C-PIB.[37] Evidently, the inherent characteristics of these Aβ radiotracers vary substantially, such as in nonspecific binding (white matter binding), range of gray matter standardized uptake values (SUVs), and discriminative ability, potentially limiting the interchangeable use of the tracers in multicenter clinical trials.[37]

In summary, great advances have been made in PET imaging of amyloids in the past 15 years, which provides several potential clinical benefits. From the clinical point of view, amyloid PET imaging offers preclinical detection of Aβ and can accurately distinguish AD from non-AD dementia in patients with mild or atypical symptoms. From the research perspective, amyloid PET imaging has allowed the investigation of the relationship (and correlation) between amyloid and cognitive function from normal aging to AD. More importantly, amyloid PET imaging, in particular with ^{11}C-PIB, has been widely used in clinical trials to monitor the biological effects of anti-Aβ drugs and has provided direct evidence for the effectiveness of these therapeutics in clearing Aβ from the brain. Unfortunately, the failure of these anti-Aβ drugs to offer cognitive and functional improvements has dampened the prospect of this approach for AD treatment.

It should be noted that most of the amyloid PET radiotracers bind mainly to fibrillary forms of Aβ. Most recently, it has been observed that ^{11}C-PIB displayed strong binding to $Aβ_{42}$ fibrils, but progressively lower binding to Arctic protofibrils and oligomers.[41] Substantial evidence has also accumulated to suggest that Aβ oligomerization and protofibril formation, rather than fibril formation, may be the more important pathogenetic event in AD. Memory impairment may be more related to the presence of soluble Aβ oligomers, which are not detectable by current amyloid PET imaging techniques. Although fibrillar forms of Aβ are thought to be in equilibrium with oligomeric forms, and they could serve as a proxy for the presence of other soluble oligomers, some healthy elderly subjects have nonetheless been found to be amyloid-positive, and some patients with MCI and or AD are amyloid-negative. As a result, amyloid PET imaging with currently available radiotracers cannot be used in isolation to make a diagnosis of AD dementia, MCI, or "normal aging." It can be used only to assess and ascertain the underlying pathophysiology of subjects who have already been clinically evaluated and given a preliminary diagnosis.

Radiotracers for Tau Protein Aggregates

In the past 2 decades, the amyloid cascade hypothesis has been the focus of AD pathogenesis, AD drug discovery, and PET imaging agent development. Indeed, the availability of amyloid radiotracers and their application in AD imaging have indicated that amyloid pathology may be a high-risk factor for future cognitive decline. However, repeated failures of clinical trials for many anti-amyloid drug candidates have recently shifted the interest to developing PET radiotracers for the tau protein aggregates, which are thought to be more closely correlated with the severity of cognitive impairment in patients with normal aging, MCI, or AD. There is also increasing evidence that at early stages of AD, neuronal toxicity is induced by soluble Aβ oligomers and tau species rather than by Aβ plaques and neurofibrillary tangles.[42]

Several tau PET tracers that share β-sheet binding properties have been reported, and tested in human studies.[43–45] Further investigations are ongoing to explore their full validation in the clinics. The chemical structures of tau PET tracers in clinical trials are depicted in **Fig. 2**.

[18]F-T807 (^{18}F-AV1451) and ^{18}F-T808

[18]F-T807 and ^{18}F-T808 displayed high affinity and selectivity for tau versus Aβ proteins in vitro. Both

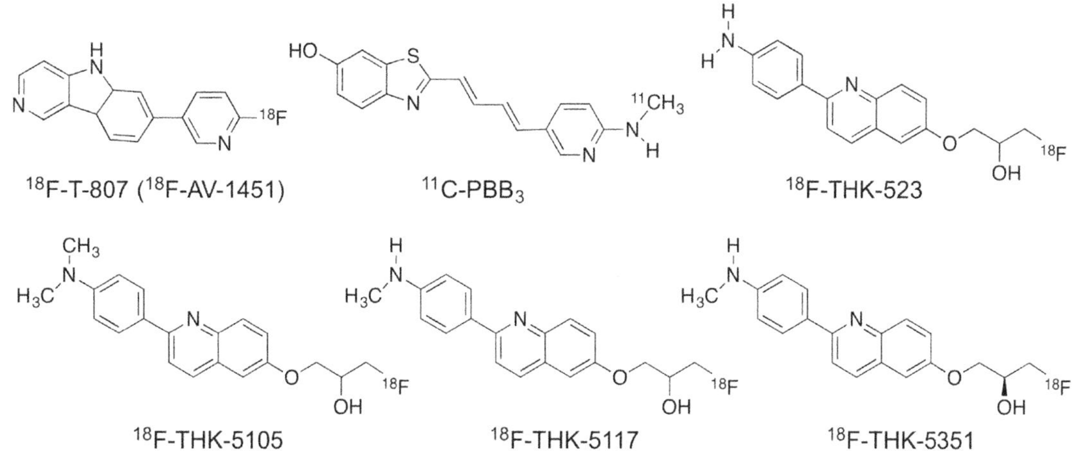

Fig. 2. Chemical structures of radiotracers for tau protein.

radiotracers exhibited favorable brain uptake and washout. However, ^{18}F-T808 had intense bone uptake in the skull due to defluorination in vivo and further clinical development was not pursued. On the other hand, ^{18}F-T807 has been shown to have overall rapid clearance from plasma and properties suitable for tau quantification with PET in human subjects. Its uptake in AD brain tracked well with expected tau pathology distribution throughout the stages of AD.[46] Most recent results favor the idea that ^{18}F-T807 binds with high affinity to tau aggregates in the form of classic paired helical filament–tau tangles containing all 6 isoforms of the tau protein (including 3R and 4R) present in AD brains and as a function of age.[47] However, it appeared to have low binding affinity to tau inclusions predominantly made of 4R isoforms that adopt a structure of straight filaments. Hence, it was suggested that ^{18}F-T807 may have limited utility for the reliable detection of tau lesions in non-AD tauopathies.[47]

[11]C-PBB3

[11]C-PBB3 displayed high specificity for tau deposits over Aβ plaques. This radiotracer has been shown to detect tau deposits in AD and non-AD tauopathies, including progressive supranuclear palsy and corticobasal degeneration.[48] However, its major radiometabolite, identified as a sulfated conjugate of ^{11}C-PBB3,[49] was shown to cross the blood-brain barrier. A recent head-to-head comparison of tau radiotracers has revealed distinct binding modes for ^{11}C-PBB3 and ^{18}F-AV1451 in brains with AD and non-AD tauopathy. Radioligand binding to brain homogenates also uncovered multiple binding components with differential affinities for ^{11}C-PBB3 and ^{18}F-AV-1451, and higher availability of binding sites on

progressive supranuclear palsy tau deposits for ^{11}C-PBB3 than ^{18}F-AV1451.[50] A cross-sectional PET study using ^{11}C-PBB3 and ^{11}C-PIB for tau and Aβ imaging, respectively, indicated a close relationship between tau accumulation and cognitive decline even in ^{11}C-PIB–negative healthy control subjects and patients with AD, but no overt relation between Aβ deposition and cognitive performance.[51]

[18]F-labeled arylquinolines (^{18}F-THK523, ^{18}F-THK5105, ^{18}F-THK5117, and ^{18}F-THK5351)

Arylquinoline derivatives were identified as lead compounds for the development of tau PET radiotracers a decade ago. ^{18}F-THK523 (^{18}F-BF242) was the first ^{18}F-labeled arylquinoline derivative; however, this tracer showed high retention in white matter and thus precluded its further use in clinical trials. Optimization of arylquinoline derivatives later led to several ^{18}F-labeled radiotracers with high selectivity for tau pathology and high retention in tau deposits in the AD brain. ^{18}F-THK5117 labeled both 3R and 4R isoforms of tau in AD brain sections. ^{18}F-THK5117 was shown to have higher signal-to-background ratio and better pharmacokinetics than ^{18}F-THK5105, and its retention was associated with dementia severity.[52] Similar to ^{18}F-THK523, ^{18}F-THK5105, and ^{18}F-THK5117 also displayed high nonspecific binding in subcortical white matter.

^{18}F-THK5351 is the S-enantiomer and pyridine derivative of ^{18}F-THK5117 with lower lipophilicity than ^{18}F-THK5117. Preclinical data demonstrated that ^{18}F-THK5351 had higher binding affinity for hippocampal homogenates from AD brains and faster dissociation from white matter than ^{18}F-THK5117, and its binding correlated with the amount of tau deposits in human brain samples.[53]

No binding to amyloid, α-synuclein, or TDP43 deposits was detected, and ^{18}F-THK5351 appeared to bind to neurofibrillary tangles with high selectivity and a higher signal-to-background ratio than ^{18}F-THK5117. Studies in mice indicated that ^{18}F-THK5351 exhibited favorable pharmacokinetics and no defluorination in vivo. In first-in-human PET imaging studies in patients with AD, ^{18}F-THK5351 demonstrated faster kinetics, higher contrast, and lower retention in subcortical white matter. A comparative study of ^{18}F-THK-5317 ([S]-^{18}F-THK5117) and ^{18}F-THK5351 showed that ^{18}F-THK5351, with prominent retention in the mesial temporal lobe and the lateral temporal cortex of patients with AD,[53] had more favorable pharmacokinetic and imaging characteristics than ^{18}F-THK5317.[54] Hence, ^{18}F-THK5351 appears to be the most promising PET radiotracer among the ^{18}F-labeled arylquinoline series for the early detection of neurofibrillary pathology in patients with AD.

Radiotracers for Neuroinflammation Biomarkers

Multiple lines of evidence have implicated neuroinflammation as one of the pathologic biomarkers in AD, and hence the neuroinflammation hypothesis of AD.[55,56] Studies have shown that, although acute inflammatory processes could protect the central nervous system against extrinsic stimuli and injuries, chronic inflammation on the other hand might be detrimental to the brain and eventually lead to its degeneration.[57,58] It is widely believed that neuroinflammation accompanies AD from its prodromal, symptom-free stage through its latest stage.[59,60] Results from both epidemiologic studies[61] and prospective clinical trials[62] have suggested that administration of nonsteroidal anti-inflammatory drugs might prevent or postpone the clinical symptoms of AD.

Neuroinflammation could be induced by either damaged neurons and neurites or pathologic protein aggregation.[63] The neuroinflammation process in AD arises from different factors, including the complement system, cytokines, growth factors, oxidative stress, microglial activation, and astrocytic reactivity.[64] These different aspects of neuroinflammation can be visualized with PET molecular probes aimed at the various targets.[65,66]

Radiotracers for the 18-kDa translocator protein

Microglia comprise 15% of the non-neuronal cells in the central nervous system. Postmortem studies revealed that activated microglia colocalize with amyloid plaques in AD brain,[67,68] suggesting that microglial activation may contribute to AD

pathology. It was later supported by experiments that under pathologic conditions such as the induction of soluble or fibrillary Aβ, microglia proliferate and release proinflammatory cytokines as well as neurotoxic substances, which eventually cause massive dysfunction and loss of neurons.[69] The 18-kDa translocator protein (TSPO), a mitochondrial protein of the microglia, is normally expressed in low levels in specific sites of the central nervous system. However, significant upregulation occurs with activation of microglia. TSPO PET tracers were thus designed to visualize microglial activity in neurologic diseases such as AD (**Fig. 3**).

^{11}C-PK11195 is the most commonly used PET radiotracer targeting TSPO. Early studies with ^{11}C-PK11195 showed significantly increased binding in the entorhinal, temporoparietal, and cingulate cortex in AD, in parallel with ^{18}F-FDG reduction in the same brain regions.[70] Multitracer PET studies using ^{11}C-PK11195 together with ^{11}C-PIB showed increased binding of both tracers in the cortical regions.[71,72] Mini Mental State Examination (MMSE) scores negatively correlated with ^{11}C-PK11195 binding but not with ^{11}C-PIB retention.[71–73] These findings suggest that microglial activation rather than Aβ as quantified by PET could parallel neuronal damage in AD. In one study, the binding of ^{11}C-PK11195 and ^{11}C-PIB negatively correlated with each other in the posterior cingulate cortex in AD,[72] suggesting that microglial activity increases at the early stage of the disease and diminishes as Aβ aggregates in the brain areas affected by AD. However, no similar correlation was found in another study in patients with MCI.[73] On the other hand, there was also evidence indicating that the alterations in ^{11}C-PK11195 binding in AD, especially at the early and prodromal stages, is too subtle to be distinguished from that in cognitively healthy controls. These studies showed that there were no significant differences between patients with AD or MCI and healthy subjects,[74,75] even if the subjects were grouped according to Aβ retention[74] or conversion to dementia from MCI.[75] There were also reports on the absence of correlation between ^{11}C-PK11195 binding and cognitive function,[75] contradicting previous results. In attempts to quantify ^{11}C-PK11195 binding more accurately, some studies applied biomathematic techniques for vascular binding[76] and reference region selection.[77]

Because the signal-to-background ratio of ^{11}C-PK11195 is relatively low, a number of ^{11}C-labeled and ^{18}F-labeled second-generation TSPO radioligands were consequently developed (see **Fig. 3**).

Neuroinflammation imaging with ^{11}C-PBR28 PET showed elevated tracer binding in multiple

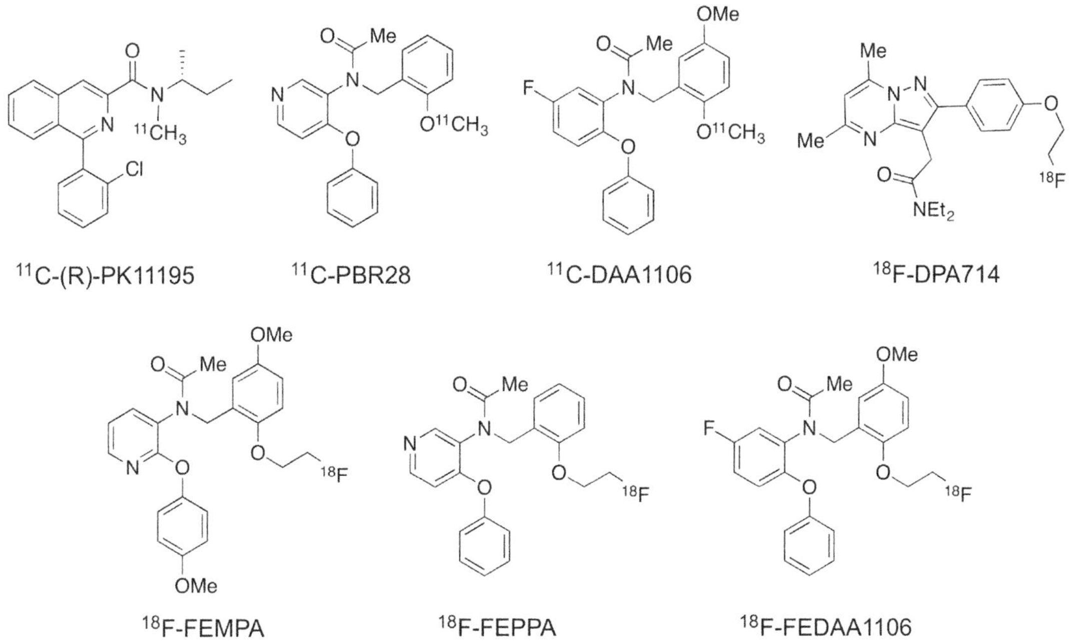

Fig. 3. Chemical structures of radiotracers for TSPO.

cortical regions in AD[78–80]; however, similar elevation pattern was not found in any brain region in patients with MCI.[78] ^{11}C-PBR28 binding had a strong positive correlation to amyloid binding as measured by ^{11}C-PIB PET and gray matter atrophy as measured by structural MR imaging.[78,79] Negative correlations were seen between TSPO binding and cognitive performances in terms of both baseline values[78] and longitudinal changes.[80] Compared with late-onset AD (LOAD), patients with early-onset AD (EOAD) showed greater binding of ^{11}C-PBR28, especially in the frontoparietal regions.[78] Meanwhile, the annual rate of increase in TSPO binding in the temporoparietal areas of MCI to AD converters were fivefold higher than nonconverters.[80] These results suggest the potential of using ^{11}C-PBR28 PET to stratify patients with AD and MCI.

[11]C-DAA1106 PET studies showed similar increased binding in cortical regions as well as striatum and cerebellum of patients with AD and MCI.[81,82] Although ^{11}C-DAA1106 binding could discriminate AD converters in MCI,[82] the severity of AD could not be assessed by ^{11}C-DAA1106 PET.[81]

One PET study with ^{18}F-DPA714 showed no difference in TSPO binding between patients with AD and healthy controls.[83] However, results from another study indicated that TSPO binding in the temporoparietal regions in patients with AD with high and mixed TSPO binding affinity were significantly greater than that in healthy controls, and was correlated with the subjects' MMSE scores and cerebral gray matter volume.[84] In the same study, ^{18}F-DPA714 binding was observed to be higher in ^{11}C-PIB–positive, cognitively healthy subjects than in ^{11}C-PIB–negative subjects, mainly in the frontal lobe. Slow cognitive decliners in AD had higher TSPO binding than fast decliners, whereas their ^{11}C-PIB PET showed no significant difference. Thus, it was suggested that microglial activation may have a neuroprotective effect at the early stages of AD.

Higher TSPO binding in AD compared with cognitively intact controls was also observed in various brain regions in PET studies using ^{18}F-FEMPA[85] and ^{18}F-FEPPA.[86] In addition, ^{18}F-FEPPA binding in the parietal cortex inversely correlated with visuospatial function, whereas binding in the posterior limb of the internal capsule inversely correlated with both visuospatial function and language ability. However, PET imaging with another ^{18}F-labeled tracer, ^{18}F-FEDAA1106, did not detect microglial activity alterations in AD.[87,88]

The disconcordant evidence relating to TSPO imaging in AD has generated multiple potential explanations. Repeated studies have shown that in addition to being activated to release proinflammatory neurotoxic substances (M1 activation), microglia could be activated (M2 activation) to release neuroprotective cytokines as well.[89] In vitro studies have shown that AD pathology may be halted with microglial inhibition.[90] What aspect of inflammation that TSPO imaging is reflecting is thus questioned by many researchers. It was also reported that TSPO is expressed in both microglia and astrocytes, which poses challenges to the quantitation of microglia activation via in vivo PET imaging, because neither first-generation nor second-generation TSPO radiotracers could well-differentiate these two types of glia, whose roles in neuroinflammation are quite the opposite.[91–94] Despite these limitations, TSPO is still the most studied target in PET imaging of neuroinflammation in AD.

Radiotracers for monoamine oxidase-B

Monoamine oxidase-B (MAO-B), an enzyme located on the outer mitochondrial membrane of astrocytes, was reported to significantly upregulate during proinflammatory processes in reactive astrocytes. Postmortem autoradiography with ^{11}C-L-deprenyl, a selective radioligand for MAO-B, demonstrated colocalization of MAO-B with plaque-associated reactive astrocytes.[95] The highest binding was observed at earliest Braak stages in AD in regions including temporal lobe and white matter, where negative correlations were found between ligand binding and Braak stages, suggesting the presence of reactive astrocytosis in early AD. This result was in line with a PET finding showing that cortical and subcortical binding of ^{11}C-deuterium-L-deprenyl (^{11}C-DED) in ^{11}C-PIB–positive patients with MCI were greater than that of healthy controls, ^{11}C-PIB–negative subjects with MCI, and patients with AD.[96] Although this study found no correlation in regional uptake of ^{11}C-DED, ^{11}C-PIB, and ^{18}F-FDG, another study found significant correlation between ^{11}C-DED and ^{11}C-PIB retention in the occipital lobe.[97]

Summary

Neuroinflammation plays an important role in the course of AD. TSPO is the most studied neuroinflammation target reflecting microglial activation, although limitations of TSPO imaging need to be overcome. For example, specific binding signal of ^{11}C-PK11195 is low, making it quite insensitive to detect changes in TSPO, whereas the second-generation TSPO radiotracers are all genotype-sensitive,[98] rendering the imaging results difficult to interpret if genotyping is not performed in study subjects. Recently, there have been efforts to develop genotype-insensitive TSPO radiotracers,[99,100] and the successful development of these radiotracers will potentially make it easier to image, quantify, and interpret TSPO imaging results in AD. In addition, radiotracers for new targets of neuroinflammation may give insights into other specific aspects of the inflammation

process. Hopefully, opposite M1/M2 activation could be specifically discriminated by using highly selective radiotracers. Future experimental designs are anticipated to focus on anti-inflammation treatment response on patients with prodromal AD with longitudinal follow-ups, and on the association of neuroinflammation biomarkers with other pathologic and pathophysiological components of AD, for example, to elucidate the time spectrum and relationship between Aβ, tau, and neuroinflammation.

PET IMAGING OF PHYSIOLOGIC BIOMARKERS IN ALZHEIMER DISEASE
Radiotracers for the Cholinergic System

Since the first description of AD more than 100 years ago, various hypotheses have been put forward in an attempt to explain AD etiology, including pathologic biomarker aggregations and pathophysiological alterations in neurotransmitter systems. Although no single-factor theory provides a satisfactory explanation for all aspects of this dementia disorder, cholinergic dysfunction was the first proposed hypothesis of its etiology, and is so far the sole basis for all the clinically approved therapeutic medications to treat AD.[101,102] It has been well-documented that cortical loss of cholinergic neurotransmission attributed to interruption of the cholinergic projections from the basal forebrain and brainstem could be the probable cause of cognitive impairment in AD.[101,103] It has also been proposed that cholinergic depletion affects neural compensatory plasticity against secondary injuries.[102] Hence, PET imaging of the cholinergic systems might provide a means to detect AD in its early stage.

PET tracers targeting components of the cholinergic system have been developed to study the in vivo pathophysiological alterations in the AD brain,[104] including those for the acetylcholinesterase (AChE) and nicotinic acetylcholine (nACh) $\alpha_4\beta_2$ and α_7 subtype receptors.

Radiotracers for acetylcholinesterase

AChE is the major therapeutic target in AD treatment to slow down cognitive deterioration, with inhibitors such as galantamine, rivastigmine, tacrine, donepezil, and memantine. AChE inhibitors increase the concentration of ACh in the synaptic cleft by inhibiting AChE hydrolysis. Autopsy evidence showed that AChE level was significantly reduced in AD brain across various neocortical regions, which strongly correlated with dementia severity.[105]

N-^{11}C-Methyl-4-piperidinyl propionate (^{11}C-PMP, **Fig. 4**) is a selective substrate for AChE

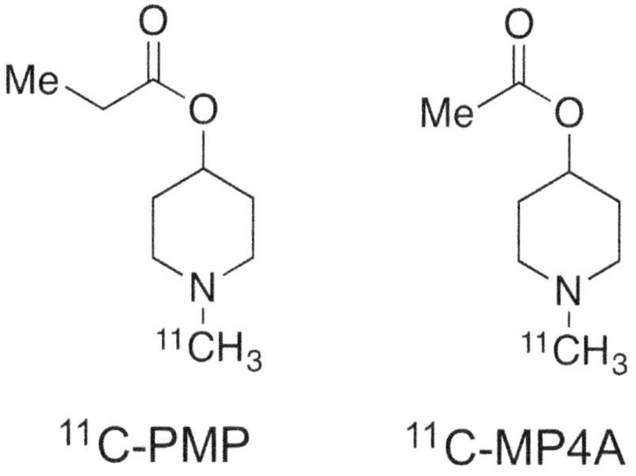

Fig. 4. Chemical structures of AChE radiotracers ^{11}C-PMP and ^{11}C-MP4A.

and has been used in PET imaging of AChE activity in AD. Kuhl and colleagues[106] found that the AChE activity was 25% to 33% lower in neocortical and hippocampal regions in patients with moderate to severe AD. The reduced activity of AChE was found to be correlated with decreased vesicular acetylcholine transporter (VAChT), as shown by 5-^{123}I-iodo-benzovesamicol (^{123}I-IBVM) single-photon emission computed tomography (SPECT), although no correlation with glucose hypometabolism was found in the posterior cingulate cortex and parietal cortex as shown by ^{18}F-FDG PET.[106] Bohnen and colleagues[107] discovered that AChE activity was modestly reduced in mild to moderate AD and that this reduction was correlated more with attention and working memory functions than with delayed short-term or long-term memory.[108] When compared with that in Parkinsonian dementia, the cortical cholinergic denervation in AD was milder,[107] and the thalamic cholinergic projection appeared not to be affected by AD.[109] The treatment effect on AChE activity in AD has also been studied using ^{11}C-PMP PET. Donepezil-induced inhibition of ^{11}C-PMP hydrolysis was found in various cortical regions, with the most inhibition in the anterior cingulate cortex, and even more pronounced inhibition in subcortical areas, such as the striatum, thalamus, and pontocerebellar regions.[110,111] The degree of cortical AChE inhibition was found to correlate with changes in executive and attentional functions but not with memory.[111] Similarly, galantamine treatment induced inhibition of cortical AChE activity in patients with AD, and the degree of inhibition correlated with attention rather than memory function.[112]

The reduction in the in vivo activity of N-^{11}C-methyl-4-piperidyl acetate (^{11}C-MP4A, see Fig. 4), another selective substrate for AChE,

was found to be more pronounced in the parieto-temporal cortex in mild AD and consistent with necropsy enzyme distribution results.[113] AChE activity in the amygdala and cerebral cortical regions was found to be significantly lower in patients with mild to moderate AD, whereas AChE activity in nucleus basalis of Meynert remained unaffected.[114] This evidence supported the hypothesis that cholinergic alterations in the neocortex and amygdala are the leading event in AD etiology. The mean cortical ^{11}C-MP4A hydrolysis rate in ApoE4-positive patients with AD was found to be significantly higher than that in ApoE4-negative patients.[115] It was therefore hypothesized that the ApoE4 allele may have a protective effect against AChE activity loss. They also found that the reduction in AChE activity correlated with word fluency task performance in ApoE noncarriers only. Donepezil and rivastigmine treatment studies using ^{11}C-MP4A PET showed similar neocortical inhibition of AChE activity in AD. The frontal inhibition, greater than its temporoparietal counterpart, was hypothesized to be associated with the behavioral and attentional improvement.[116,117]

Radiotracers for nicotinic acetylcholine receptors

Postmortem studies showed that nicotinic acetylcholine receptors (nAChRs) rather than muscarinic receptors were profoundly affected in AD.[118,119] ^{11}C-Nicotine (Fig. 5), a nonselective radioligand for nAChRs, was the first to be used in the investigation of nAChRs in AD. Cortical reduction of ^{11}C-nicotine binding was observed in early PET studies of patients with AD.[120,121] Attention test and visuospatial ability test results correlated with ^{11}C-nicotine binding both globally and regionally. However, no significant correlation was observed between episodic memory test results and ^{11}C-nicotine binding in any brain region.[122] Similar to AChE PET results, alterations in ^{11}C-nicotine binding after galantamine treatment were found to correlate significantly with attention but not to episodic memory.[112]

2-^{18}F-F-A-85380 (^{18}F-2FA, see Fig. 5) is a selective radiotracer for the $\alpha_4\beta_2$ subtype of nAChR. Ellis and colleagues[123] observed a significant negative correlation between the attention task results and frontal ^{18}F-2FA distribution volume in early AD, although it was suggested that ^{18}F-2FA PET may be insensitive to differentiate patients with early AD from age-matched healthy controls. In contrast, studies conducted by other groups found significant reduction in $\alpha_4\beta_2$ nAChR distribution volume in patients with early to severe AD and patients with amnestic MCI.[124–126] These studies also found significant correlations between [18]F-2FA binding in the AD-affected regions and multiple cognitive functions. Notably, [18]F-2FA binding potential in patients with MCI that converted to AD later on was found to be further reduced compared with that of patients with stable MCI.[125] A significant correlation was also found between ^{11}C-PIB binding in the frontal cortex and [18]F-2FA binding in the medial frontal cortex and nucleus basalis magnocellularis, suggesting a contribution of amyloid toxicity to the dysfunction of cholinergic system.[126] Contrary to what was found in AChE PET studies, galantamine induced no significant changes in cortical [18]F-2FA binding. In addition, no correlation was found between $\alpha_4\beta_2$ nAChR binding and cognitive test results in terms of either absolute value or percentage changes.[127]

The tissue kinetics of [18]F-2FA is slow, and PET imaging requires a long scanning time, which poses a challenge to patients with AD. Recently, a new generation of $\alpha_4\beta_2$ nAChR PET radiotracers with faster tissue kinetic has been developed.[128,129] Two of these radiotracers, ^{18}F-AZAN and (−)-^{18}F-flubatine (also known as [−]-^{18}F-NCFHEB) (see **Fig. 5**), have been advanced to human use.[130,131] Using a bolus plus constant infusion protocol of radiotracer administration, binding parameters of (−)-^{18}F-flubatine could be reliably calculated with 30 minutes of scan data, which will make it easier to use in patients with challenging disorders such as AD.[132]

The α_7 subtype of nAChR is also believed to play an important role in AD pathophysiology, as it binds to $A\beta_{1-42}$ with high affinity, mediates $A\beta$-induced tau phosphorylation, and contributes to neuronal cell death.[133,134] α_7 nAChR agonists inhibit this binding and prevent $A\beta_{1-42}$-induced toxicity.[135] In addition, α_7 nAChR is also expressed on microglia and astrocytes and is involved in AD-associated neuroinflammation and neurodegeneration.[136,137] Hence, the α_7 nAChR appears to be a prime target in AD investigation. However, there have been no suitable radiotracers for PET imaging of the α_7 nAChR in humans until recently, when ^{18}F-ASEM and ^{18}F-DBT-10 (see **Fig. 5**), 2 regioisomers of the same chemical formula, were discovered to provide adequate α_7-specific binding signals in nonhuman primates.[138–141] ^{18}F-ASEM has since been advanced to human use, and PET scans of 90 minutes' duration were shown to be sufficient to quantify α_7 nAChR binding parameters in healthy subjects.[138,142] Its application in AD imaging will provide additional insights into the roles of α_7 nAChR in AD pathogenesis and progression, and the effectiveness of α_7 nAChR agonists in AD treatment.

Summary

Cholinergic dysfunction plays a critical role in AD. Current PET imaging with various cholinergic biomarkers has revealed the connection between cholinergic dysfunction and AD. Because current clinically approved treatments are focusing mainly on the AChE system, cholinergic PET might be helpful for screening drug-sensitive/insensitive candidates, and could help to monitor treatment response. Further research, especially longitudinal,

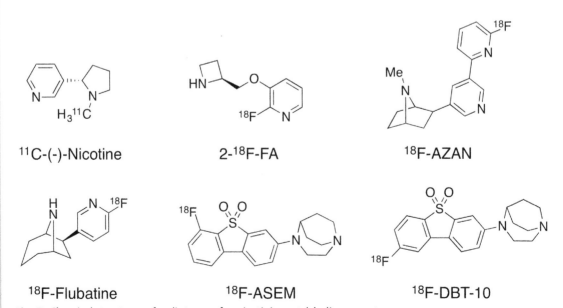

^{11}C-(-)-Nicotine   2-^{18}F-FA ^{18}F-AZAN

^{18}F-Flubatine ^{18}F-ASEM ^{18}F-DBT-10

Fig. 5. Chemical structures of radiotracers for nicotinic acetylcholine receptors.

multiprobe imaging studies of large hierarchical populations, are expected to focus on disease progression, therapeutic response to AD medications, and association with other pathologic and pathophysiological aspects of the disease.

Imaging of Neuronal Activity in Alzheimer Disease with ^{18}F-Fluorodeoxyglucose

The major metabolic substrate used in human brain is glucose, whose radiolabeled analogue ^{18}F-fluoro-2-deoxy-D-glucose (^{18}F-FDG) is the most widely used PET radiotracer, with the first ^{18}F-FDG PET application in human brain imaging.[143] ^{18}F-FDG uptake in the cerebral cortices are closely related to cytoarchitectonic structure and synaptic function,[144] whose alteration occurs before neuronal death and perceivable atrophy.

In terms of functional imaging of AD, ^{18}F-FDG PET is usually conducted for early detection and to predict cognitive decline in AD, and to differentiate AD from other dementing neurodegenerative disorders, such as vascular dementia, dementia of Lewy bodies (DLB), and frontotemporal dementia (FTD). Here, we review clinical ^{18}F-FDG PET studies focusing on AD dementia and its prodromal stage.

^{18}F-Fluorodeoxyglucose PET manifestation in Alzheimer disease dementia

The most prominent characteristic of ^{18}F-FDG PET in AD dementia is decreased glucose metabolism in the parietotemporal association regions as well as the posterior cingulate cortex and precuneus.[145] The latter regions are absent in typical presentation of other cognition disorders such as DLB, enabling them to be sensitive biomarkers in terms of clinical differentiation. The temporal lobe is another region that is frequently affected by AD. Reduction of glucose metabolism in the frontal lobe is usually observed in later-stage AD cases, although this phenomenon is also seen in normal aging.

In contrast, regions including sensorimotor cortex, visual cortex, and basal ganglia are often unaffected in AD.[146] Hippocampal hypometabolism is thought to be present in the early stages of AD[147]; however, its identification is not easily done through visual inspection, and depends mainly on software-based comparison when targeted regional analyses are applied.[148] In most cases, specific clinical symptoms could be related to topographic hypometabolism seen in the individual ^{18}F-FDG PET images. For instance, speech comprehension disability is associated with hypometabolism in the Wernicke area, whereas facial recognition impairment is associated with hypometabolism in the fusiform gyrus.[149]

EOAD, defined by the clinical onset of AD before the age of 65 years, is characterized by the tendency to progress more rapidly compared with LOAD, with clinical onset later than the age of 65 years. Growing evidence suggests that the hypometabolic pattern of EOAD could be different from that of LOAD. In contrast to LOAD, hypometabolism in EOAD is more severe[24,150] and more asymmetric, especially in the left precuneus and left supramarginal gyrus.[151] Decreases in ^{18}F-FDG metabolic connectivity centered in the cingulate and occipital cortex were seen in EOAD, whereas connectivity decreases were localized in different regions in LOAD. The connectivity between these EOAD regions was correlated with disease severity and clinical dementia rating scores. Global efficiency and clustering coefficients were decreased in EOAD rather than in LOAD and were also correlated to disease severity.[152] Patients with EOAD exhibited poorer executive function and greater parietal hypometabolism, whereas patients with LOAD presented poorer confrontation naming and verbal recognition memories and greater hypometabolism in the inferior frontotemporal cortices.[153] It was hypothesized that early parietal-frontal network disturbance might be present in EOAD, because executive deficits were not consistent with frontal hypometabolism. Behavioral abnormalities were associated with cerebral metabolic alterations in EOAD. Hyperactivity and affective subsyndromes and apathetic subsyndrome in patients with EOAD were significantly correlated with regional hypermetabolism and hypometabolism, respectively, in various frontal regions.[154]

Voxelwise statistical software using various computational techniques have been developed to aid differentiation of dementia categories and subcategories. In a study comparing the diagnostic accuracy and confidence of physicians differentiating AD/MCI, DLB, and FTD, 43% of the overall cases had a corrected misdiagnosis or improved diagnostic confidence for the correct diagnosis when applying 3-dimensional stereotactic surface projection in addition to standard visual inspection.[155] The efficacy of automated discrimination using AD image statistics (t-sum: sum of t statistics) was tested in large sample databases of Alzheimer's Disease Neuroimaging Initiative (ADNI) and Network for Standardisation of Dementia Diagnosis (NEST-DD).[156] It was found that the t-sum of patients with AD was significantly higher than that of healthy controls, and was correlated with severity of dementia. This automated method provided good discriminating power with a sensitivity and specificity of 83% and 78%, respectively, in the ADNI group and of 78% and 94%, respectively, in the NEST-DD group. In addition, the AD t-sum of EOAD was found to be higher than that of LOAD, consistent with the differences in their clinical characteristics.

18F-Fluorodeoxyglucose PET manifestation in prodromal Alzheimer disease

Amnestic MCI was considered to be the prodromal stage of AD dementia. In view of the failure of various therapeutic clinical trials targeting the AD population with dementia, functional neuroimaging studies are focusing on screening of patients with prodromal AD in an attempt to prevent or delay their onset of dementia. ^{18}F-FDG PET seeks to find correlation between cerebral metabolic alterations of these patients and their neuropsychiatric symptoms, and to predict whether and when the patient would eventually convert to AD dementia.[157]

In MCI, hypometabolism in the inferior parietal lobe, precuneus, and posterior cingulate cortex, the same hypometabolic regions as found in AD dementia, were thought to have dementia-conversion predicting ability. In a meta-analysis comparing the accuracy of ^{18}F-FDG PET, cerebral blood flow (CBF) SPECT and structural MR imaging for predicting short-term conversion from MCI to AD dementia,[158] the sensitivity and specificity of ^{18}F-FDG PET (88.8% and 84.9%, respectively) were higher than those of CBF SPECT (83.8% and 70.4%, respectively) and structural MR imaging (72.8% and 81%, respectively). In another meta-analysis estimating the diagnostic accuracy of ^{18}F-FDG PET and ^{11}C-PIB PET for predicting the conversion from MCI to AD dementia,[159] ^{18}F-FDG PET was shown to have a higher specificity (74.0% vs 56.2%) but a lower sensitivity (78.7% vs 93.5%) compared with ^{11}C-PIB PET. It is hypothesized that the relatively preserved cerebral synaptic function, as indicated by ^{18}F-FDG metabolism, demonstrates compensatory mechanisms against the neural amyloid burden as demonstrated by ^{11}C-PIB PET. Combined clinical information with ^{18}F-FDG PET, MR imaging, and cerebrospinal fluid (CSF) markers provided the highest accuracy for predicting MCI conversion, as compared with using only one or two of the biomarkers.[160] ^{18}F-FDG PET contributed the most in all the components, especially when ApoE4 genotype and cognitive testing information were available.

Relative hypermetabolism in the occipital lobe was also observed in amnestic MCI, especially in those subjects free of amyloid burden.[161] This assumed compensation of glucose metabolism in the early phase of the disease against synaptic dysfunction in the parietotemporal association cortex was thought to contribute to the nonconversion of the subjects in comparison with their hypometabolic counterparts.

18F-Fluorodeoxyglucose PET monitoring treatment response in Alzheimer disease

There have been several clinical studies using ^{18}F-FDG PET to monitor treatment response in AD. A significant increase of glucose metabolism in the left dorsolateral frontoparietal network and bilateral temporal cortex was observed in AD brain after receiving metrifonate treatment,[162] and a global increase was observed following memantine treatment.[163] Compared with nonresponders and placebo receivers, responders presented increased hippocampal and prefrontal metabolism after rivastigmine treatment.[164]

Summary

^{18}F-FDG PET is a widely applied and useful tool in diagnosis and treatment monitoring in AD. It is especially valuable in the differentiation of AD from other dementing disorders, as well as in the prediction of MCI conversion. Longitudinal follow-up studies are ongoing in multiple centers.

Radiotracers for Imaging of Synaptic Density in Alzheimer's Disease

The loss of synapses is a consistent and robust pathology in AD.[165–167] Synapses are essential for cognitive function, and cognitive impairment is closely associated with the loss of synapses in AD.[6,166,168–170] Reductions in synapses are already present in the neocortex and limbic system during MCI, a prodromal form of AD or other dementias.[5,171,172] The exact sequence of molecular events that lead to synaptic damage and neurodegeneration are not yet fully understood. Accumulation of toxic Aβ oligomers is believed to be related to loss of synapses and presynaptic proteins in patients with MCI,[5–7,173] but more recent research also suggests an emerging role for tau-mediated toxicity at the synapse.[174,175]

Synaptic density can be quantified in brain tissue using electron microscopy; however, this method is typically time-consuming and technically demanding. An alternative, indirect measurement of synapses has relied on quantification of synaptic markers, typically proteins located in high abundance in close proximity to synapses. Light or confocal microscopy imaging combined with immunohistochemistry has focused on imaging of proteins related to secretory vesicles. Synaptic vesicle proteins are prime biomarker candidates based on the restricted cellular localization of vesicles in synaptic boutons, their ubiquitous distribution in the brain, and high phylogenic conservation across vertebrate nervous systems.[176–179] One of the most established synaptic markers is synaptophysin, one of the first characterized[178,180] and cloned,[181] as well as most abundant synaptic vesicle protein.[182] In vivo quantification of synaptic density in the living brain may thus be possible with PET imaging in combination with a synapse-specific radioligand.

Very recently, several PET radioligands have been developed for imaging of synaptic vesicle glycoprotein 2A (SV2A).[183] Synaptic vesicle glycoprotein 2 (SV2) is an integral glycoprotein located in the cell membrane of secretory vesicles,[184,185] and is the molecular target of the antiepileptic drug levetiracetam.[186] There are three known SV2 protein isoforms, SV2A, SV2B, and SV2C, with SV2A as the isoform ubiquitously and homogeneously located in synapses across the brain.[187–189] SV2B is found throughout the brain, but in a more restricted distribution than SV2A. SV2C has been observed in a few brain regions, including the globus pallidus, substantia nigra, midbrain, brainstem, and olfactory bulb.[187–189] Thus, PET imaging of SV2A could be an excellent in vivo proxy biomarker for synaptic density.

To date, 4 SV2A PET radioligands have been reported in the literature, including ^{11}C-levetiracetam, ^{11}C-UCB-A, ^{18}F-UCB-H, and ^{11}C-UCB-J (**Fig. 6**).[190–193] Radiosynthesis of ^{11}C-levetiracetam was shown to be feasible with a multiple-step scheme, but its in vivo evaluation has not been reported so far. It is, however, likely that the SV2A affinity of levetiracetam ($K_i = 1.6$ µM) is too low to render ^{11}C-levetiracetam a useful PET radioligand.[192,194] ^{11}C-UCB-A has been characterized in the brain of rats and pigs and was found to bind specifically to SV2A. Binding kinetics of ^{11}C-UCB-A is, however, slow in both species, possibly related to the slow metabolism and clearance of the tracer.[190] The first ^{18}F-labeled radioligand, ^{18}F-UCB-H, has been more extensively investigated, including studies in rats and humans. The binding of ^{18}F-UCB-H was shown to be specific to SV2A in rats,[195] and radiation dosimetry was found acceptable in rodents and humans.[193,196] More recently, an improved radiosynthesis method has been described,[197] but in vivo characterization of this radioligand in the human brain has not yet been reported.[193,195–197] Finally, an extensive evaluation of ^{11}C-UCB-J has been reported, and this radioligand currently appears to be the most promising for quantification of SV2A in the human brain.[191,198]

[11]C-UCB-J was demonstrated to exhibit excellent characteristics as an SV2A PET radioligand in rhesus macaques, including high brain uptake and fast kinetics.[191] Binding specificity of ^{11}C-UCB-J to SV2A was confirmed in blocking and displacement experiments with administration of SV2A agent levetiracetam or brivaracetam.[191,199] Analyses of monkey plasma and rat brain tissue indicated that the circulating radiolabeled metabolites are polar and thus not likely to cross the blood-brain barrier. In comparison, ^{11}C-UCB-J displayed significantly higher specific binding than ^{18}F-UCB-H in the nonhuman primate brain.[191]

In a follow-up study, SV2A was confirmed to be a valid alternative synaptic density marker to synaptophysin.[198] After a PET scan with ^{11}C-UCB-J, a baboon was euthanized and brain tissues were sampled for analyses by Western blotting, confocal microscopy, and SV2A homogenate binding assays. The results from these studies demonstrated an excellent linear correlation between SV2A and the "gold standard" synaptic marker synaptophysin across all gray matter regions, and considerable overlap in the cellular distribution of SV2A and synaptophysin in the cortex. Furthermore, the in vitro regional distribution of SV2A correlated well with the in vivo ^{11}C-UCB-J binding as measured by PET imaging.

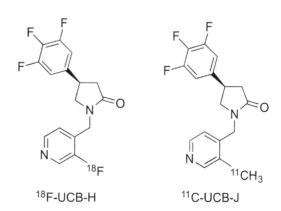

[11]C-Levetiracetam   ^{11}C-UCB-A   ^{18}F-UCB-H   ^{11}C-UCB-J

Fig. 6. Chemical structures of radiotracers for SV2A.

The pharmacokinetic and imaging properties of ^{11}C-UCB-J were then evaluated in healthy human subjects.[198] Similar to nonhuman primates, high radioactivity concentrations (SUV of 7–11) were observed in all gray matter regions while uptake in white matter regions was low. ^{11}C-UCB-J displayed favorable kinetics suitable for quantification by using the 1-tissue compartment model, and regional distribution volume (V_T) values could be reliably estimated with a scan duration as short as 60 minutes. Quantification of ^{11}C-UCB-J was shown to be highly reliable, with low test-retest and intersubject variability in regional V_T values.[198,200] Similar to the results in nonhuman primates, binding of ^{11}C-UCB-J in humans was displaceable by the anticonvulsant levetiracetam.[198]

The white matter region centrum semiovale is being considered as a potential reference region for the quantification of nondisplaceable ^{11}C-UCB-J binding. In an extensive in vitro examination of baboon brain tissue, it was confirmed that SV2A density was negligible in the white matter.[198] However, a small apparent reduction in V_T was observed in the centrum semiovale of human subjects after administration of levetiracetam.[198] Further validation studies with SV2A elective inhibitors, for example, levetiracetam or brivaracetam, are ongoing at the Yale PET Center to confirm the promise of a reference region approach for quantification of ^{11}C-UCB-J binding.

To evaluate the sensitivity of SV2A PET to synaptic loss, ^{11}C-UCB-J binding was evaluated in 3 patients with temporal lobe epilepsy and mesial temporal sclerosis.[198] In all subjects, there was a decreased uptake (~52% asymmetry in BP_{ND}) in the hippocampus ipsilateral to the mesial temporal sclerosis seen on MR imaging. Preliminarily, ^{11}C-UCB-J binding has also been found to be decreased in the brain of patients with AD, with highest reductions in the hippocampus (**Fig. 7**).

In summary, PET imaging of SV2A is a promising biomarker strategy for quantification of synaptic density in the human brain. Validation studies in animals and humans have been performed and demonstrated that the SV2A radioligand ^{11}C-UCB-J is sensitive to detect synaptic loss in patients with epilepsy and AD. PET imaging of synaptic density is a promising approach for research, clinical diagnosis, and therapeutic monitoring in AD, and other neurologic disorders in which synaptic disruption and/or loss are indicated.

PERSPECTIVES

AD is a progressive, complex neurologic disorder involving multiple pathophysiological processes, from loss of synaptic density and neuronal loss, to neuroinflammation, to deposition of β-amyloid plaques and neurofibrillary tangles, and resulting in the progressive impairment of cognitive functions and memory loss. Early diagnosis is the key to effectively treat the disease before manifestation of clinical symptoms.

In the past two decades, PET imaging agents targeting various pathologic and physiologic biomarkers in AD has made great contributions to the investigation and diagnosis of this disease. In particular, the development of Aβ imaging agents has allowed the differentiation of AD and non-AD dementia, the tracking of Aβ burden along the temporal progression of the disease, the stratification of patients for clinical trials of anti-Aβ drugs, and the monitoring of biological effects of such therapeutic agents. Results from PET imaging of Aβ burden in moderate to severe AD have been found to largely parallel glucose hypometabolism as imaged by ^{18}F-FDG. However, findings in healthy elderly subjects and patients with MCI are more variable, and correlation with ^{18}F-FDG hypometabolism and cognitive function is relatively weak. Hence, whether Aβ imaging alone will have predictive value in early AD diagnosis remains to be proven.

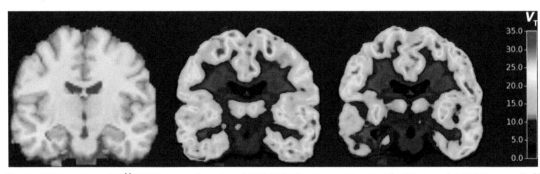

Fig. 7. PET imaging with ^{11}C-UCB-J reveals reduced SV2A binding in a patient with AD. Template MR image (*left*) and corresponding volume of distribution (V_T) maps of ^{11}C-UCB-J in one elder control (*middle*, 74-year-old man) and one patient with AD (*right*, 82-year-old man).

Radiotracers for the other pathologic hallmark of AD, tau protein aggregates, are in the early phase of clinical evaluation. Their value in the early diagnosis and progression monitoring of disease will become clear as more data become available.

PET imaging agents targeting other pathologic and physiologic biomarkers of AD, such as the neuroinflammation biomarker TSPO, cholinergic receptors, and the synaptic protein SV2A, are also available for use in AD imaging. As cholinergic dysfunction, synaptic loss, and microglial activation have all been thought to precede the formation of neurofibrillary tangles in AD, application of PET radiotracers for these targets, together with those for Aβ and tau, in multimodal imaging studies, will help unravel the topographic progression of different pathologic and physiologic biomarkers, shed new lights on AD etiology and progression, and identify the most appropriate biomarker for truly early diagnosis of AD. Measurement of synaptic density through PET imaging of the synaptic biomarker SV2A may hold particular promise in this regard and be able to detect cognitive abnormalities in the prodromal and preclinical stages, as loss of synaptic density has been shown to be closely correlated with cognitive impairment. This, of course, will need to be proven in large-scale clinical trials of the SV2A imaging agent in healthy elderly subjects, subjects with MCI, and patients with AD.

REFERENCES

1. Querfurth HW, LaFerla FM. Alzheimer's disease. N Engl J Med 2010;362(4):329–44.
2. Goedert M, Spillantini MG. A century of Alzheimer's disease. Science 2006;314(5800):777–81.
3. Holtzman DM, John CM, Goate A. Alzheimer's disease: the challenge of the second century. Sci Transl Med 2011;3(77):77sr1.
4. Jack CR Jr, Albert MS, Knopman DS, et al. Introduction to the recommendations from the National Institute on Aging-Alzheimer's Association workgroups on diagnostic guidelines for Alzheimer's disease. Alzheimers Dement 2011;7(3):257–62.
5. Pham E, Crews L, Ubhi K, et al. Progressive accumulation of amyloid-β oligomers in Alzheimer's disease and in amyloid precursor protein transgenic mice is accompanied by selective alterations in synaptic scaffold proteins. FEBS J 2010;277(14):3051–67.
6. Robinson JL, Molina-Porcel L, Corrada MM, et al. Perforant path synaptic loss correlates with cognitive impairment and Alzheimer's disease in the oldest-old. Brain 2014;137(Pt 9):2578–87.
7. Beeri MS, Haroutunian V, Schmeidler J, et al. Synaptic protein deficits are associated with dementia irrespective of extreme old age. Neurobiol Aging 2012;33(6):1125.e1-8.
8. Shankar G, Walsh D. Alzheimer's disease: synaptic dysfunction and abeta. Mol Neurodegener 2009; 4(1):48.
9. McKhann GM, Knopman DS, Chertkow H, et al. The diagnosis of dementia due to Alzheimer's disease: recommendations from the National Institute on Aging-Alzheimer's Association workgroups on diagnostic guidelines for Alzheimer's disease. Alzheimers Dement 2011;7(3):263–9.
10. Hardy JA, Higgins GA. Alzheimer's disease: the amyloid cascade hypothesis. Science 1992;256:184–5.
11. Hardy J, Allsop D. Amyloid deposition as the central event in the aetiology of Alzheimer's disease. Trends Pharmacol Sci 1991;12(10):383–8.
12. Hardy J, Duff K, Hardy KG, et al. Genetic dissection of Alzheimer's disease and related dementias: amyloid and its relationship to tau. Nat Neurosci 1998;1(5):355–8.
13. Vallabhajosula S. Positron emission tomography radiopharmaceuticals for imaging brain β-amyloid. Semin Nucl Med 2011;41(4):283–99.
14. Mathis CA, Mason NS, Lopresti BJ, et al. Development of positron emission tomography β-amyloid plaque imaging agents. Semin Nucl Med 2012; 42(6):423–32.
15. Cselenyi Z, Jönhagen ME, Forsberg A, et al. Clinical validation of ^{18}F-AZD4694, an amyloid-β-specific PET radioligand. J Nucl Med 2012;53(3):415–24.
16. Rowe CC, Pejoska S, Mulligan RS, et al. Head-to-head comparison of ^{11}C-PiB and ^{18}F-AZD4694 (NAV4694) for β-amyloid imaging in aging and dementia. J Nucl Med 2013;54(6):880–6.
17. Klunk WE, Engler H, Nordberg A, et al. Imaging brain amyloid in Alzheimer's disease with Pittsburgh compound-B. Ann Neurol 2004;55(3):306–19.
18. Cohen AD. Using Pittsburgh compound B for PET imaging across the Alzheimer's disease spectrum. Technology Innovation 2016;18(1):51–61.
19. Rowe CC, Villemagne VL. Brain amyloid imaging. J Nucl Med 2011;52(11):1733–40.
20. Forsberg A, Engler H, Almkvist O, et al. PET imaging of amyloid deposition in patients with mild cognitive impairment. Neurobiol Aging 2008; 29(10):1456–65.
21. Kemppainen NM, Scheinin NM, Koivunen J, et al. Five-year follow-up of ^{11}C-PIB uptake in Alzheimer's disease and MCI. Eur J Nucl Med Mol Imaging 2014;41(2):283–9.
22. Koivunen J, Scheinin N, Virta JR, et al. Amyloid PET imaging in patients with mild cognitive impairment: a 2-year follow-up study. Neurology 2011;76(12): 1085–90.
23. Villemagne VL, Pike KE, Chételat G, et al. Longitudinal assessment of Aβ and cognition in aging and Alzheimer disease. Ann Neurol 2011;69(1):181–92.

24. Bahar-Fuchs A, Villemagne V, Ong K, et al. Prediction of amyloid-β pathology in amnestic mild cognitive impairment with neuropsychological tests. J Alzheimers Dis 2013;33(2):451–62.

25. Albert MS, DeKosky ST, Dickson D, et al. The diagnosis of mild cognitive impairment due to Alzheimer's disease: recommendations from the National Institute on Aging-Alzheimer's Association workgroups on diagnostic guidelines for Alzheimer's disease. Alzheimers Dement 2011;7(3):270–9.

26. Klunk WE. Amyloid imaging as a biomarker for cerebral beta-amyloidosis and risk prediction for Alzheimer dementia. Neurobiol Aging 2011;32(Suppl 1):S20–36.

27. Grundman M, Pontecorvo MJ, Salloway SP, et al. Potential impact of amyloid imaging on diagnosis and intended management in patients with progressive cognitive decline. Alzheimer Dis Assoc Disord 2013;27(1):4–15.

28. Boccardi M, Altomare D, Ferrari C, et al. Assessment of the incremental diagnostic value of florbetapir F-18 imaging in patients with cognitive impairment: the incremental diagnostic value of Amyloid PET with [18F]-Florbetapir (India-FBP) Study. JAMA Neurol 2016;73(12):1417–24.

29. Syed YY, Deeks E. [18F]Florbetaben: a review in β-Amyloid PET imaging in cognitive impairment. CNS Drugs 2015;29(7):605–13.

30. Daerr S, Brendel M, Zach C, et al. Evaluation of early-phase [18F]-florbetaben PET acquisition in clinical routine cases. Neuroimage Clin 2017;14:77–86.

31. Ikonomovic MD, Buckley CJ, Heurling K, et al. Post-mortem histopathology underlying β-amyloid PET imaging following flutemetamol F-18 injection. Acta Neuropathol Commun 2016;4(1):130.

32. Beach TG, Thal DR, Zanette M, et al. Detection of striatal amyloid plaques with [18F]flutemetamol: validation with postmortem histopathology. J Alzheimers Dis 2016;52(3):863–73.

33. Zwan MD, Bouwman FH, Konijnenberg E, et al. Diagnostic impact of [18F]flutemetamol PET in early-onset dementia. Alzheimers Res Ther 2017;9(1):2.

34. Bensaidane MR, Beauregard JM, Poulin S, et al. Clinical utility of amyloid PET Imaging in the differential diagnosis of atypical dementias and its impact on caregivers. J Alzheimers Dis 2016;52(4):1251–62.

35. Rowe CC, Jones G, Doré V, et al. Standardized expression of 18F-NAV4694 and 11C-PiB β-Amyloid PET results with the centiloid scale. J Nucl Med 2016;57(8):1233–7.

36. Klunk WE, Koeppe RA, Price JC, et al. The centiloid project: standardizing quantitative amyloid plaque estimation by PET. Alzheimers Dement 2015; 11(1):1–15.e1-4.

37. Chiotis K, Carter SF, Farid K, et al. Amyloid PET in European and North American cohorts; and exploring age as a limit to clinical use of amyloid imaging. Eur J Nucl Med Mol Imaging 2015; 42(10):1492–506.

38. Morris E, Chalkidou A, Hammers A, et al. Diagnostic accuracy of 18F amyloid PET tracers for the diagnosis of Alzheimer's disease: a systematic review and meta-analysis. Eur J Nucl Med Mol Imaging 2016;43(2):374–85.

39. Johnson KA, Minoshima S, Bohnen NI, et al. Appropriate use criteria for amyloid PET: a report of the amyloid imaging task force, the society of nuclear medicine and molecular imaging, and the Alzheimer's association. Alzheimers Dement 2013; 9(1):e-1-16.

40. Johnson KA, Minoshima S, Bohnen NI, et al. Update on appropriate use criteria for amyloid PET imaging: dementia experts, mild cognitive impairment, and education. Amyloid imaging task force of the Alzheimer's Association and Society for Nuclear Medicine and Molecular Imaging. Alzheimers Dement 2013;9(4):e106–9.

41. Yamin G, Teplow DB. Pittsburgh compound-B (PiB) binds amyloid β-protein protofibrils. J Neurochem 2017;140(2):210–5.

42. Gotz J, Ittner LM. Animal models of Alzheimer's disease and frontotemporal dementia. Nat Rev Neurosci 2008;9(7):532–44.

43. Shah M, Catafau AM. Molecular imaging insights into neurodegeneration: focus on tau PET radiotracers. J Nucl Med 2014;55(6):871–4.

44. Okamura N, Harada R, Furumoto S, et al. Tau PET imaging in Alzheimer's disease. Curr Neurol Neurosci Rep 2014;14(11):500.

45. Harada R, Okamura N, Furumoto S, et al. Characteristics of tau and its ligands in PET imaging. Biomolecules 2016;6(1):7.

46. Wooten D, Guehl NJ, Verwer EE, et al. Pharmacokinetic evaluation of the tau PET radiotracer [18F] T807 ([18F]AV-1451) in human subjects. J Nucl Med 2017;58(3):484–91.

47. Marquie M, Normandin MD, Meltzer AC, et al. Pathological correlations of [F-18]-AV-1451 imaging in non-Alzheimer tauopathies. Ann Neurol 2017; 81(1):117–28.

48. Maruyama M, Shimada H, Suhara T, et al. Imaging of tau pathology in a tauopathy mouse model and in Alzheimer patients compared to normal controls. Neuron 2013;79(6):1094–108.

49. Hashimoto H, Kawamura K, Takei M, et al. Identification of a major radiometabolite of [11C]PBB3. Nucl Med Biol 2015;42(12):905–10.

50. Ono M, Sahara N, Kumata K, et al. Distinct binding of PET ligands PBB3 and AV-1451 to tau fibril strains in neurodegenerative tauopathies. Brain 2017;140(3):764–80.

51. Shimada H, Kitamura S, Shinotoh H, et al. Association between Aβ and tau accumulations and their influence on clinical features in aging and Alzheimer's disease spectrum brains: a [11C]PBB3-PET study. Alzheimers Dement (Amst) 2017;6:11–20.

52. Harada R, Okamura N, Furumoto S, et al. [18F]THK-5117 PET for assessing neurofibrillary pathology in Alzheimer's disease. Eur J Nucl Med Mol Imaging 2015;42:1052–61.

53. Harada R, Okamura N, Furumoto S, et al. 18F-THK5351: a novel PET radiotracer for imaging neurofibrillary pathology in Alzheimer disease. J Nucl Med 2016;57(2):208–14.

54. Betthauser T, Lao PJ, Murali D, et al. In vivo comparison of tau radioligands 18F-THK-5351 and 18F-THK-5317. J Nucl Med 2017. [Epub ahead of print].

55. McGeer EG, McGeer PL. Neuroinflammation in Alzheimer's disease and mild cognitive impairment: a field in its infancy. J Alzheimer's Dis 2010;19(1): 355–61.

56. Morales I, Guzman-Martinez L, Cerda-Troncoso C, et al. Neuroinflammation in the pathogenesis of Alzheimer's disease. A rational framework for the search of novel therapeutic approaches. Front Cell Neurosci 2014;8:112.

57. Wyss-Coray T, Mucke L. Inflammation in neurodegenerative disease–a double-edged sword. Neuron 2002;35(3):419–32.

58. Mrak RE, Griffin WS. Glia and their cytokines in progression of neurodegeneration. Neurobiol Aging 2005;26(3):349–54.

59. Vehmas AK, Kawas CH, Stewart WF, et al. Immune reactive cells in senile plaques and cognitive decline in Alzheimer's disease. Neurobiol Aging 2003;24(2):321–31.

60. Hoozemans JJ, van Haastert ES, Veerhuis R, et al. Maximal COX-2 and ppRb expression in neurons occurs during early Braak stages prior to the maximal activation of astrocytes and microglia in Alzheimer's disease. J Neuroinflammation 2005;2:27.

61. McGeer PL, Schulzer M, McGeer EG. Arthritis and anti-inflammatory agents as possible protective factors for Alzheimer's disease: a review of 17 epidemiologic studies. Neurology 1996;47(2):425–32.

62. Hoozemans JJ, Veerhuis R, Rozemuller JM, et al. Soothing the inflamed brain: effect of nonsteroidal anti-inflammatory drugs on Alzheimer's disease pathology. CNS Neurol Disord Drug Targets 2011;10(1):57–67.

63. Barger SW, Harmon AD. Microglial activation by Alzheimer amyloid precursor protein and modulation by apolipoprotein E. Nature 1997;388(6645): 878–81.

64. Akiyama H, Barger S, Barnum S, et al. Inflammation and Alzheimer's disease. Neurobiol Aging 2000; 21(3):383–421.

65. Zimmer ER, Leuzy A, Benedet AL, et al. Tracking neuroinflammation in Alzheimer's disease: the role of positron emission tomography imaging. J Neuroinflammation 2014;11:120.

66. Varley J, Brooks DJ, Edison P. Imaging neuroinflammation in Alzheimer's disease and other dementias: recent advances and future directions. Alzheimers Dement 2015;11(9):1110–20.

67. McGeer PL, Itagaki S, Boyes BE, et al. Reactive microglia are positive for HLA-DR in the substantia nigra of Parkinson's and Alzheimer's disease brains. Neurology 1988;38(8):1285–91.

68. Venneti S, Lopresti BJ, Wang G, et al. PK11195 labels activated microglia in Alzheimer's disease and in vivo in a mouse model using PET. Neurobiol Aging 2009;30(8):1217–26.

69. Schilling T, Eder C. Amyloid-beta-induced reactive oxygen species production and priming are differentially regulated by ion channels in microglia. J Cell Physiol 2011;226(12):3295–302.

70. Cagnin A, Brooks DJ, Kennedy AM, et al. In-vivo measurement of activated microglia in dementia. Lancet 2001;358(9280):461–7.

71. Edison P, Archer HA, Gerhard A, et al. Microglia, amyloid, and cognition in Alzheimer's disease: an [11C]-(R)-PK11195-PET and [11C]PIB-PET study. Neurobiol Dis 2008;32(3):412–9.

72. Yokokura M, Mori N, Yagi S, et al. In vivo changes in microglial activation and amyloid deposits in brain regions with hypometabolism in Alzheimer's disease. Eur J Nucl Med Mol Imaging 2011;38(2): 343–51.

73. Okello A, Edison P, Archer HA, et al. Microglial activation and amyloid deposition in mild cognitive impairment: a PET study. Neurology 2009;72(1): 56–62.

74. Wiley CA, Lopresti BJ, Venneti S, et al. Carbon 11-labeled Pittsburgh Compound B and carbon 11-labeled (R)-PK11195 positron emission tomographic imaging in Alzheimer disease. Arch Neurol 2009;66(1):60–7.

75. Schuitemaker A, Kropholler MA, Boellaard R, et al. Microglial activation in Alzheimer's disease: an (R)-[11C]PK11195 positron emission tomography study. Neurobiol Aging 2013;34(1):128–36.

76. Tomasi G, Edison P, Bertoldo A, et al. Novel reference region model reveals increased microglial and reduced vascular binding of 11C-(R)-PK11195 in patients with Alzheimer's disease. J Nucl Med 2008;49(8):1249–56.

77. Yaqub M, van Berckel BN, Schuitemaker A, et al. Optimization of supervised cluster analysis for extracting reference tissue input curves in (R)-[11C] PK11195 brain PET studies. J Cereb Blood Flow Metab 2012;32(8):1600–8.

78. Kreisl WC, Lyoo CH, McGwier M, et al. In vivo radioligand binding to translocator protein correlates

with severity of Alzheimer's disease. Brain 2013; 136(Pt 7):2228–38.

79. Kreisl WC, Lyoo CH, Liow JS, et al. Distinct patterns of increased translocator protein in posterior cortical atrophy and amnestic Alzheimer's disease. Neurobiol Aging 2016;51:132–40.

80. Kreisl WC, Lyoo CH, Liow JS, et al. ^{11}C-PBR28 binding to translocator protein increases with progression of Alzheimer's disease. Neurobiol Aging 2016;44:53–61.

81. Yasuno F, Ota M, Kosaka J, et al. Increased binding of peripheral benzodiazepine receptor in Alzheimer's disease measured by positron emission tomography with ^{11}C]DAA1106. Biol Psychiatry 2008;64(10):835–41.

82. Yasuno F, Kosaka J, Ota M, et al. Increased binding of peripheral benzodiazepine receptor in mild cognitive impairment-dementia converters measured by positron emission tomography with ^{11}C]DAA1106. Psychiatry Res 2012;203(1):67–74.

83. Golla SS, Boellaard R, Oikonen V, et al. Quantification of ^{18}F]DPA-714 binding in the human brain: initial studies in healthy controls and Alzheimer's disease patients. J Cereb Blood Flow Metab 2015;35(5):766–72.

84. Hamelin L, Lagarde J, Dorothée G, et al. Early and protective microglial activation in Alzheimer's disease: a prospective study using ^{18}F-DPA-714 PET imaging. Brain 2016;139(Pt 4):1252–64.

85. Varrone A, Oikonen V, Forsberg A, et al. Positron emission tomography imaging of the 18-kDa translocator protein (TSPO) with ^{18}F]FEMPA in Alzheimer's disease patients and control subjects. Eur J Nucl Med Mol Imaging 2015;42(3):438–46.

86. Suridjan I, Pollock BG, Verhoeff NP, et al. In-vivo imaging of grey and white matter neuroinflammation in Alzheimer's disease: a positron emission tomography study with a novel radioligand, ^{18}F]-FEPPA. Mol Psychiatry 2015;20(12):1579–87.

87. Varrone A, Mattsson P, Forsberg A, et al. In vivo imaging of the 18-kDa translocator protein (TSPO) with ^{18}F]FEDAA1106 and PET does not show increased binding in Alzheimer's disease patients. Eur J Nucl Med Mol Imaging 2013;40(6):921–31.

88. Gulyas B, Vas A, Tóth M, et al. Age and disease related changes in the translocator protein (TSPO) system in the human brain: positron emission tomography measurements with ^{11}C]vinpocetine. Neuroimage 2011;56(3):1111–21.

89. Mosser DM, Edwards JP. Exploring the full spectrum of macrophage activation. Nat Rev Immunol 2008;8(12):958–69.

90. Prokop S, Miller KR, Heppner FL. Microglia actions in Alzheimer's disease. Acta Neuropathol 2013; 126(4):461–77.

91. Rojas S, Martín A, Arranz MJ, et al. Imaging brain inflammation with ^{11}C]PK11195 by PET and induction of the peripheral-type benzodiazepine receptor after transient focal ischemia in rats. J Cereb Blood Flow Metab 2007;27(12):1975–86.

92. Ji B, Maeda J, Sawada M, et al. Imaging of peripheral benzodiazepine receptor expression as biomarkers of detrimental versus beneficial glial responses in mouse models of Alzheimer's and other CNS pathologies. J Neurosci 2008;28(47):12255–67.

93. Venneti S, Wang G, Nguyen J, et al. The positron emission tomography ligand DAA1106 binds with high affinity to activated microglia in human neurological disorders. J Neuropathol Exp Neurol 2008; 67(10):1001–10.

94. Lavisse S, Guillermier M, Hérard AS, et al. Reactive astrocytes overexpress TSPO and are detected by TSPO positron emission tomography imaging. J Neurosci 2012;32(32):10809–18.

95. Gulyas B, Pavlova E, Kása P, et al. Activated MAO-B in the brain of Alzheimer patients, demonstrated by ^{11}C]-L-deprenyl using whole hemisphere autoradiography. Neurochem Int 2011; 58(1):60–8.

96. Carter SF, Schöll M, Almkvist O, et al. Evidence for astrocytosis in prodromal Alzheimer disease provided by ^{11}C-deuterium-L-deprenyl: a multitracer PET paradigm combining ^{11}C-Pittsburgh compound B and ^{18}F-FDG. J Nucl Med 2012;53(1): 37–46.

97. Santillo AF, Gambini JP, Lannfelt L, et al. In vivo imaging of astrocytosis in Alzheimer's disease: an ^{11}C-L-deuteriodeprenyl and PIB PET study. Eur J Nucl Med Mol Imaging 2011;38(12):2202–8.

98. Owen DR, Matthews PM. Imaging brain microglial activation using positron emission tomography and translocator protein-specific radioligands. Int Rev Neurobiol 2011;101:19–39.

99. Zanotti-Fregonara P, Zhang Y, Jenko KJ, et al. Synthesis and evaluation of translocator 18 kDa protein (TSPO) positron emission tomography (PET) radioligands with low binding sensitivity to human single nucleotide polymorphism rs6971. ACS Chem Neurosci 2014;5(10):963–71.

100. Ikawa M, Lohith TG, Shrestha S, et al. ^{11}C-ER176, a radioligand for 18-kDa translocator protein, has adequate sensitivity to robustly image all three affinity genotypes in human brain. J Nucl Med 2017;58(2):320–5.

101. Bartus RT, Dean RL 3rd, Beer B, et al. The cholinergic hypothesis of geriatric memory dysfunction. Science 1982;217(4558):408–14.

102. Craig LA, Hong NS, McDonald RJ. Revisiting the cholinergic hypothesis in the development of Alzheimer's disease. Neurosci Biobehav Rev 2011; 35(6):1397–409.

103. Schliebs R, Arendt T. The cholinergic system in aging and neuronal degeneration. Behav Brain Res 2011;221(2):555–63.

104. Roy R, Niccolini F, Pagano G, et al. Cholinergic imaging in dementia spectrum disorders. Eur J Nucl Med Mol Imaging 2016;43(7):1376–86.

105. Bierer LM, Haroutunian V, Gabriel S, et al. Neurochemical correlates of dementia severity in Alzheimer's disease: relative importance of the cholinergic deficits. J Neurochem 1995;64(2): 749–60.

106. Kuhl DE, Koeppe RA, Minoshima S, et al. In vivo mapping of cerebral acetylcholinesterase activity in aging and Alzheimer's disease. Neurology 1999;52(4):691–9.

107. Bohnen NI, Kaufer DI, Ivanco LS, et al. Cortical cholinergic function is more severely affected in parkinsonian dementia than in Alzheimer disease: an in vivo positron emission tomographic study. Arch Neurol 2003;60(12):1745–8.

108. Bohnen NI, Kaufer DI, Hendrickson R, et al. Cognitive correlates of cortical cholinergic denervation in Parkinson's disease and parkinsonian dementia. J Neurol 2006;253(2):242–7.

109. Kotagal V, Muller ML, Kaufer DI, et al. Thalamic cholinergic innervation is spared in Alzheimer disease compared to parkinsonian disorders. Neurosci Lett 2012;514(2):169–72.

110. Kuhl DE, Minoshima S, Frey KA, et al. Limited donepezil inhibition of acetylcholinesterase measured with positron emission tomography in living Alzheimer cerebral cortex. Ann Neurol 2000;48(3): 391–5.

111. Bohnen NI, Kaufer DI, Hendrickson R, et al. Degree of inhibition of cortical acetylcholinesterase activity and cognitive effects by donepezil treatment in Alzheimer's disease. J Neurol Neurosurg Psychiatry 2005;76(3):315–9.

112. Kadir A, Darreh-Shori T, Almkvist O, et al. PET imaging of the in vivo brain acetylcholinesterase activity and nicotine binding in galantamine-treated patients with AD. Neurobiol Aging 2008;29(8): 1204–17.

113. Iyo M, Namba H, Fukushi K, et al. Measurement of acetylcholinesterase by positron emission tomography in the brains of healthy controls and patients with Alzheimer's disease. Lancet 1997;349(9068): 1805–9.

114. Herholz K, Weisenbach S, Zündorf G, et al. In vivo study of acetylcholine esterase in basal forebrain, amygdala, and cortex in mild to moderate Alzheimer disease. Neuroimage 2004;21(1):136–43.

115. Eggers C, Herholz K, Kalbe E, et al. Cortical acetylcholine esterase activity and ApoE4-genotype in Alzheimer disease. Neurosci Lett 2006;408(1): 46–50.

116. Shinotoh H, Aotsuka A, Fukushi K, et al. Effect of donepezil on brain acetylcholinesterase activity in patients with AD measured by PET. Neurology 2001;56(3):408–10.

117. Kaasinen V, Någren K, Järvenpää T, et al. Regional effects of donepezil and rivastigmine on cortical acetylcholinesterase activity in Alzheimer's disease. J Clin Psychopharmacol 2002;22(6):615–20.

118. Flynn DD, Mash DC. Characterization of L-[^{3}H] nicotine binding in human cerebral cortex: comparison between Alzheimer's disease and the normal. J Neurochem 1986;47(6):1948–54.

119. Sabbagh MN, Shah F, Reid RT, et al. Pathologic and nicotinic receptor binding differences between mild cognitive impairment, Alzheimer disease, and normal aging. Arch Neurol 2006;63(12):1771–6.

120. Nordberg A, Hartvig P, Lilja A, et al. Decreased uptake and binding of ^{11}C-nicotine in brain of Alzheimer patients as visualized by positron emission tomography. J Neural Transm Park Dis Dement Sect 1990;2(3):215–24.

121. Nordberg A, Lundqvist H, Hartvig P, et al. Kinetic analysis of regional (S)-^{11}C-nicotine binding in normal and Alzheimer brains–in vivo assessment using positron emission tomography. Alzheimer Dis Assoc Disord 1995;9(1):21–7.

122. Kadir A, Almkvist O, Wall A, et al. PET imaging of cortical ^{11}C-nicotine binding correlates with the cognitive function of attention in Alzheimer's disease. Psychopharmacology (Berl) 2006;188(4):509–20.

123. Ellis JR, Villemagne VL, Nathan PJ, et al. Relationship between nicotinic receptors and cognitive function in early Alzheimer's disease: a 2-[^{18}F]fluoro-A-85380 PET study. Neurobiol Learn Mem 2008;90(2):404–12.

124. Sabri O, Kendziorra K, Wolf H, et al. Acetylcholine receptors in dementia and mild cognitive impairment. Eur J Nucl Med Mol Imaging 2008; 35(Suppl 1):S30–45.

125. Kendziorra K, Wolf H, Meyer PM, et al. Decreased cerebral α4β2* nicotinic acetylcholine receptor availability in patients with mild cognitive impairment and Alzheimer's disease assessed with positron emission tomography. Eur J Nucl Med Mol Imaging 2011;38(3):515–25.

126. Okada H, Ouchi Y, Ogawa M, et al. Alterations in alpha4beta2 nicotinic receptors in cognitive decline in Alzheimer's aetiopathology. Brain 2013; 136(Pt 10):3004–17.

127. Ellis JR, Nathan PJ, Villemagne VL, et al. Galantamine-induced improvements in cognitive function are not related to alterations in $\alpha_4\beta_2$ nicotinic receptors in early Alzheimer's disease as measured in vivo by 2-[^{18}F]fluoro-A-85380 PET. Psychopharmacology (Berl) 2009;202(1–3): 79–91.

128. Horti AG, Gao Y, Kuwabara H, et al. Development of radioligands with optimized imaging properties for quantification of nicotinic acetylcholine receptors by positron emission tomography. Life Sci 2010;86(15–16):575–84.

129. Meyer PM, Tiepolt S, Barthel H, et al. Radioligand imaging of α4β2* nicotinic acetylcholine receptors in Alzheimer's disease and Parkinson's disease. Q J Nucl Med Mol Imaging 2014;58(4):376–86.

130. Wong DF, Kuwabara H, Kim J, et al. PET imaging of high-affinity α4β2 nicotinic acetylcholine receptors in humans with ^{18}F-AZAN, a radioligand with optimal brain kinetics. J Nucl Med 2013;54(8):1308–14.

131. Sabri O, Becker GA, Meyer PM, et al. First-in-human PET quantification study of cerebral α4β2* nicotinic acetylcholine receptors using the novel specific radioligand (−)-[^{18}F]Flubatine. Neuroimage 2015;118:199–208.

132. Hillmer AT, Esterlis I, Gallezot JD, et al. Imaging of cerebral $\alpha_4\beta_2^*$ nicotinic acetylcholine receptors with (−)-[^{18}F]Flubatine PET: implementation of bolus plus constant infusion and sensitivity to acetylcholine in human brain. Neuroimage 2016; 141:71–80.

133. Wang HY, Lee DH, D'Andrea MR, et al. β-Amyloid1–42 binds to α7 nicotinic acetylcholine receptor with high affinity. Implications for Alzheimer's disease pathology. J Biol Chem 2000;275(8): 5626–32.

134. Wang HY, Li W, Benedetti NJ, et al. α7 nicotinic acetylcholine receptors mediate beta-amyloid peptide-induced tau protein phosphorylation. J Biol Chem 2003;278(34):31547–53.

135. Buckingham SD, Jones AK, Brown LA, et al. Nicotinic acetylcholine receptor signalling: roles in Alzheimer's disease and amyloid neuroprotection. Pharmacol Rev 2009;61(1):39–61.

136. Conejero-Goldberg C, Davies P, Ulloa L. Alpha7 nicotinic acetylcholine receptor: a link between inflammation and neurodegeneration. Neurosci Biobehav Rev 2008;32(4):693–706.

137. Wang H, Yu M, Ochani M, et al. Nicotinic acetylcholine receptor α7 subunit is an essential regulator of inflammation. Nature 2003;421(6921):384–8.

138. Hillmer AT, Li S, Zheng MQ, et al. PET imaging of α7 nicotinic acetylcholine receptors: a comparative study of [^{18}F]ASEM and [^{18}F]DBT-10 in nonhuman primates, and further evaluation of [^{18}F]ASEM in humans. Eur J Nucl Med Mol Imaging 2017. [Epub ahead of print].

139. Hillmer AT, Zheng MQ, Li S, et al. PET imaging evaluation of [^{18}F]DBT-10, a novel radioligand specific to alpha7 nicotinic acetylcholine receptors, in nonhuman primates. Eur J Nucl Med Mol Imaging 2016;43(3):537–47.

140. Horti AG. Development of [^{18}F]ASEM, a specific radiotracer for quantification of the alpha7-nAChR with positron-emission tomography. Biochem Pharmacol 2015;97(4):566–75.

141. Horti AG, Gao Y, Kuwabara H, et al. ^{18}F-ASEM, a radiolabeled antagonist for imaging the alpha7-nicotinic acetylcholine receptor with PET. J Nucl Med 2014;55(4):672–7.

142. Wong DF, Kuwabara H, Pomper M, et al. Human brain imaging of α7 nAChR with [^{18}F]ASEM: a new PET radiotracer for neuropsychiatry and determination of drug occupancy. Mol Imaging Biol 2014;16(5):730–8.

143. Phelps ME, Huang SC, Hoffman EJ, et al. Tomographic measurement of local cerebral glucose metabolic rate in humans with (F-18)2-fluoro-2-deoxy-D-glucose: validation of method. Ann Neurol 1979;6(5):371–88.

144. Sokoloff L. The deoxyglucose method for the measurement of local glucose utilization and the mapping of local functional activity in the central nervous system. Int Rev Neurobiol 1981;22:287–333.

145. Minoshima S, Frey KA, Koeppe RA, et al. A diagnostic approach in Alzheimer's disease using three-dimensional stereotactic surface projections of fluorine-18-FDG PET. J Nucl Med 1995; 36(7):1238–48.

146. Pascual B, Prieto E, Arbizu J, et al. Brain glucose metabolism in vascular white matter disease with dementia: differentiation from Alzheimer disease. Stroke 2010;41(12):2889–93.

147. Mosconi L, Mistur R, Switalski R, et al. FDG-PET changes in brain glucose metabolism from normal cognition to pathologically verified Alzheimer's disease. Eur J Nucl Med Mol Imaging 2009;36(5): 811–22.

148. Mosconi L, Tsui WH, De Santi S, et al. Reduced hippocampal metabolism in MCI and AD: automated FDG-PET image analysis. Neurology 2005;64(11): 1860–7.

149. Herholz K. Guidance for reading FDG PET scans in dementia patients. Q J Nucl Med Mol Imaging 2014;58(4):332–43.

150. Sakamoto S, Ishii K, Sasaki M, et al. Differences in cerebral metabolic impairment between early and late onset types of Alzheimer's disease. J Neurol Sci 2002;200(1–2):27–32.

151. Chiaravalloti A, Koch G, Toniolo S, et al. Comparison between early-onset and late-onset Alzheimer's disease patients with amnestic presentation: CSF and ^{18}F-FDG PET Study. Dement Geriatr Cogn Dis Extra 2016;6(1):108–19.

152. Chung J, Yoo K, Kim E, et al. Glucose metabolic brain networks in early-onset vs. late-onset Alzheimer's disease. Front Aging Neurosci 2016;8:159.

153. Kaiser NC, Melrose RJ, Liu C, et al. Neuropsychological and neuroimaging markers in early versus late-onset Alzheimer's disease. Am J Alzheimers Dis Other Demen 2012;27(7):520–9.

154. Ballarini T, Iaccarino L, Magnani G, et al. Neuropsychiatric subsyndromes and brain metabolic network dysfunctions in early onset Alzheimer's disease. Hum Brain Mapp 2016;37(12):4234–47.

155. Kim J, Cho SG, Song M, et al. Usefulness of 3-dimensional stereotactic surface projection FDG PET images for the diagnosis of dementia. Medicine (Baltimore) 2016;95(49):e5622.

156. Haense C, Herholz K, Jagust WJ, et al. Performance of FDG PET for detection of Alzheimer's disease in two independent multicentre samples (NEST-DD and ADNI). Dement Geriatr Cogn Disord 2009;28(3):259–66.

157. Ito K, Fukuyama H, Senda M, et al. Prediction of outcomes in mild cognitive impairment by using ^{18}F-FDG-PET: a multicenter study. J Alzheimer's Dis 2015;45(2):543–52.

158. Yuan Y, Gu ZX, Wei WS. Fluorodeoxyglucose-positron-emission tomography, single-photon emission tomography, and structural MR imaging for prediction of rapid conversion to Alzheimer disease in patients with mild cognitive impairment: a meta-analysis. AJNR Am J Neuroradiol 2009;30(2):404–10.

159. Zhang S, Han D, Tan X, et al. Diagnostic accuracy of ^{18}F-FDG and ^{11}C-PIB-PET for prediction of short-term conversion to Alzheimer's disease in subjects with mild cognitive impairment. Int J Clin Pract 2012;66(2):185–98.

160. Shaffer JL, Petrella JR, Sheldon FC, et al. Predicting cognitive decline in subjects at risk for Alzheimer disease by using combined cerebrospinal fluid, MR imaging, and PET biomarkers. Radiology 2013;266(2):583–91.

161. Ashraf A, Fan Z, Brooks DJ, et al. Cortical hypermetabolism in MCI subjects: a compensatory mechanism? Eur J Nucl Med Mol Imaging 2015; 42(3):447–58.

162. Mega MS, Cummings JL, O'Connor SM, et al. Cognitive and metabolic responses to metrifonate therapy in Alzheimer disease. Neuropsychiatry Neuropsychol Behav Neurol 2001;14(1):63–8.

163. Schmidt R, Ropele S, Pendl B, et al. Longitudinal multimodal imaging in mild to moderate Alzheimer disease: a pilot study with memantine. J Neurol Neurosurg Psychiatry 2008;79(12):1312–7.

164. Potkin SG, Anand R, Fleming K, et al. Brain metabolic and clinical effects of rivastigmine in Alzheimer's disease. Int J Neuropsychopharmacol 2001;4(3):223–30.

165. Scheff SW, DeKosky ST, Price DA. Quantitative assessment of cortical synaptic density in Alzheimer's disease. Neurobiol Aging 1990;11(1):29–37.

166. Terry RD, Masliah E, Salmon DP, et al. Physical basis of cognitive alterations in Alzheimer's disease: synapse loss is the major correlate of cognitive impairment. Ann Neurol 1991;30(4):572–80.

167. Scheff SW, Price DA. Alzheimer's disease-related alterations in synaptic density: neocortex and hippocampus. J Alzheimers Dis 2006;9(3 Suppl): 101–15.

168. DeKosky ST, Scheff SW. Synapse loss in frontal cortex biopsies in Alzheimer's disease: correlation with cognitive severity. Ann Neurol 1990;27(5):457–64.

169. DeKosky ST, Scheff SW, Styren SD. Structural correlates of cognition in dementia: quantification and assessment of synapse change. Neurodegeneration 1996;5(4):417–21.

170. Hamos JE, DeGennaro LJ, Drachman DA. Synaptic loss in Alzheimer's disease and other dementias. Neurology 1989;39(3):355–61.

171. Masliah E, Mallory M, Alford M, et al. Altered expression of synaptic proteins occurs early during progression of Alzheimer's disease. Neurology 2001;56(1):127–9.

172. Masliah E, Mallory M, Hansen L, et al. Synaptic and neuritic alterations during the progression of Alzheimer's disease. Neurosci Lett 1994;174(1):67–72.

173. Wei W, Nguyen LN, Kessels HW, et al. Amyloid beta from axons and dendrites reduces local spine number and plasticity. Nat Neurosci 2010;13(2): 190–6.

174. Pooler AM, Noble W, Hanger DP. A role for tau at the synapse in Alzheimer's disease pathogenesis. Neuropharmacology 2014;76 Pt A:1–8.

175. Wang Y, Mandelkow E. Tau in physiology and pathology. Nat Rev Neurosci 2016;17(1):5–21.

176. Goelz SE, Nestler EJ, Chehrazi B, et al. Distribution of protein I in mammalian brain as determined by a detergent-based radioimmunoassay. Proc Natl Acad Sci U S A 1981;78(4):2130–4.

177. Perdahl E, Adolfsson R, Alafuzoff I, et al. Synapsin I (protein I) in different brain regions in senile dementia of Alzheimer type and in multi-infarct dementia. J Neural Transm 1984;60(2):133–41.

178. Navone F, Jahn R, Di Gioia G, et al. Protein p38: an integral membrane protein specific for small vesicles of neurons and neuroendocrine cells. J Cell Biol 1986;103(6 Pt 1):2511–27.

179. De Camilli P, Harris SM Jr, Huttner WB, et al. Synapsin I (Protein I), a nerve terminal-specific phosphoprotein. II. Its specific association with synaptic vesicles demonstrated by immunocytochemistry in agarose-embedded synaptosomes. J Cell Biol 1983;96(5):1355–73.

180. Wiedenmann B, Franke WW. Identification and localization of synaptophysin, an integral membrane glycoprotein of Mr 38,000 characteristic of presynaptic vesicles. Cell 1985;41(3):1017–28.

181. Leube RE, Kaiser P, Seiter A, et al. Synaptophysin: molecular organization and mRNA expression as determined from cloned cDNA. EMBO J 1987; 6(11):3261–8.

182. Takamori S, Holt M, Stenius K, et al. Molecular anatomy of a trafficking organelle. Cell 2006;127(4): 831–46.

183. Mercier J, Archen L, Bollu V, et al. Discovery of heterocyclic nonacetamide synaptic vesicle protein

2A (SV2A) ligands with single-digit nanomolar potency: opening avenues towards the first SV2A positron emission tomography (PET) ligands. ChemMedChem 2014;9(4):693–8.

184. Bajjalieh SM, Peterson K, Shinghal R, et al. SV2, a brain synaptic vesicle protein homologous to bacterial transporters. Science 1992;257(5074): 1271–3.

185. Feany MB, Lee S, Edwards RH, et al. The synaptic vesicle protein SV2 is a novel type of transmembrane transporter. Cell 1992;70(5):861–7.

186. Lynch BA, Lambeng N, Nocka K, et al. The synaptic vesicle protein SV2A is the binding site for the antiepileptic drug levetiracetam. Proc Natl Acad Sci U S A 2004;101(26):9861–6.

187. Janz R, Sudhof TC. SV2C is a synaptic vesicle protein with an unusually restricted localization: anatomy of a synaptic vesicle protein family. Neuroscience 1999;94(4):1279–90.

188. Bajjalieh SM, Frantz GD, Weimann JM, et al. Differential expression of synaptic vesicle protein 2 (SV2) isoforms. J Neurosci 1994;14(9):5223–35.

189. Bajjalieh SM, Peterson K, Linial M, et al. Brain contains two forms of synaptic vesicle protein 2. Proc Natl Acad Sci U S A 1993;90(6):2150–4.

190. Estrada S, Lubberink M, Thibblin A, et al. [^{11}C] UCB-A, a novel PET tracer for synaptic vesicle protein 2A. Nucl Med Biol 2016;43(6):325–32.

191. Nabulsi NB, Mercier J, Holden D, et al. Synthesis and preclinical evaluation of ^{11}C-UCB-J as a PET tracer for imaging the synaptic vesicle glycoprotein 2A in the brain. J Nucl Med 2016;57(5):777–84.

192. Cai H, Mangner TJ, Muzik O, et al. Radiosynthesis of ^{11}C-levetiracetam: a potential marker for PET imaging of SV2A expression. ACS Med Chem Lett 2014;5(10):1152–5.

193. Bretin F, Warnock G, Bahri MA, et al. Preclinical radiation dosimetry for the novel SV2A radiotracer [^{18}F]UCB-H. EJNMMI Res 2013;3(1):35.

194. Gillard M, Chatelain P, Fuks B. Binding characteristics of levetiracetam to synaptic vesicle protein 2A (SV2A) in human brain and in CHO cells expressing the human recombinant protein. Eur J Pharmacol 2006;536(1–2):102–8.

195. Warnock GI, Aerts J, Bahri MA, et al. Evaluation of ^{18}F-UCB-H as a novel PET tracer for synaptic vesicle protein 2A in the brain. J Nucl Med 2014; 55(8):1336–41.

196. Bretin F, Bahri MA, Bernard C, et al. Biodistribution and radiation dosimetry for the novel SV2A radiotracer [^{18}F]UCB-H: first-in-human study. Mol Imaging Biol 2015;17(4):557–64.

197. Warnier C, Lemaire C, Becker G, et al. Enabling efficient positron emission tomography (PET) imaging of synaptic vesicle glycoprotein 2A (SV2A) with a robust and one-step radiosynthesis of a highly potent ^{18}F-labeled ligand ([^{18}F]UCB-H). J Med Chem 2016;59(19):8955–66.

198. Finnema SJ, Nabulsi NB, Eid T, et al. Imaging synaptic density in the living human brain. Sci Transl Med 2016;8(348):348ra96.

199. Nicolas JM, Hannestad J, Holden D, et al. Brivaracetam, a selective high-affinity synaptic vesicle protein 2A (SV2A) ligand with preclinical evidence of high brain permeability and fast onset of action. Epilepsia 2016;57(2):201–9.

200. Finnema S, Nabulsi N, Mercier J, et al. [C-11]UCB-J is a suitable PET tracer for imaging of synaptic vesicle glycoprotein 2A (SV2A) in humans. J Nucl Med 2015;56(Suppl 3):249.

Multimodal PET Imaging of Amyloid and Tau Pathology in Alzheimer Disease and Non–Alzheimer Disease Dementias

Chenjie Xia, MD[a], Bradford C. Dickerson, MD[b],*

KEYWORDS

• Alzheimer disease • Dementia • Amyloid PET imaging • Tau PET imaging • Biomarker

KEY POINTS

• Amyloid PET imaging is a crucial biomarker for accurate diagnosis and therapy development for Alzheimer disease (AD).
• Tau PET imaging will complement amyloid PET imaging for AD and serve as a valuable biomarker for non-AD tauopathies, such as frontotemporal lobar degeneration (FTLD).
• Molecular PET imaging can allow examining longitudinal progression of amyloid and tau pathology in individuals who are cognitively normal or who have mild cognitive impairment (MCI) to better understand risk factors for and transition to dementia.
• Multimodal studies, including amyloid and tau PET imaging, will allow examining how molecular pathologies interact with other markers of neural integrity, such as glucose metabolism (fluorodeoxyglucose [FDG]-PET), functional connectivity or task-related activation (functional MR imaging), and gray and white matter structural integrity (structural MR imaging or diffusion tensor imaging).

WHY IS THERE A NEED FOR PATHOLOGY-SPECIFIC MOLECULAR PET IMAGING?

Traditionally, the diagnosis of AD and non-AD dementias (eg, frontotemporal dementia [FTD], primary progressive aphasia [PPA], and parkinsonian dementias) has primarily relied on characterizing clinical phenotypes through a detailed evaluation, which includes history taking, mental status, and neurologic examination, often supplemented by neuropsychological evaluation. This process often leads a clinician to understand that a patient's clinical phenotype matches one of several broad categories defined by the predominant cognitive domain affected, such as memory, executive function, language, visuospatial function, or socioaffective function, with each pointing to a specific associated clinical diagnosis. For example, a patient presenting with progressive episodic memory deficits is most likely to have probable AD, whereas a patient presenting with

Disclosure Statement: Dr B.C. Dickerson has received consulting fees from Merck and Piramal. Dr C. Xia has nothing to disclose.
[a] Department of Neurology, Jewish General Hospital, McGill University, 3755 Chemin de la Côte-Sainte-Catherine Road, Suite E-005, Montreal, QC H3T 1E2, Canada; [b] Frontotemporal Disorders Unit, Department of Neurology, Massachusetts General Hospital, Harvard University, 149 13th Street, Suite 2691, Charlestown, Boston, MA 02129, USA
* Corresponding author.
E-mail address: brad.dickerson@mgh.harvard.edu

PET Clin 12 (2017) 351–359
http://dx.doi.org/10.1016/j.cpet.2017.02.005
1556-8598/17/© 2017 Elsevier Inc. All rights reserved.

progressive language impairments is most likely to have PPA. In some patients, characteristic motor abnormalities, such as parkinsonism or motor neuron disease features, can also offer valuable diagnostic clues. A patient presenting with executive dysfunction, visuospatial impairment, visual hallucinations, and parkinsonism is likely to receive a diagnosis of dementia with Lewy bodies (DLB).

After this formulation of the most likely clinical syndrome based on predominant clinical symptoms, clinicians turn toward imaging, most often structural MR imaging. Characteristic cortical atrophy patterns seen on a T1-weighted MR image can also strengthen the original diagnostic hypothesis, such as medial temporal lobe atrophy seen in AD dementia or temporal pole atrophy seen in the semantic variant of PPA. In some settings, FDG-PET is used in a similar fashion—to support the clinical hypothesis regarding the localization of neurodegeneration. This culminates in a clinical diagnosis of AD, FTD, DLB, or another condition that is probabilistically associated with the underlying pathology or pathologies most often underlying that condition. In some cases, this clinical diagnosis with supportive MR imaging or FDG-PET findings is highly predictive of underlying pathology. For example, in a patient with clinically typical semantic variant PPA[1] or progressive supranuclear palsy (PSP), the pathology is highly likely to be TDP-43 or tau-PSP, respectively. In contrast, 10% to 20% of individuals diagnosed with clinically typical AD exhibit non-AD pathologies. And a patient diagnosed with the behavioral variant of FTD is nearly equally likely to exhibit tau or TDP-43 pathology.[2] The term FTD is used to indicate the clinical dementia syndrome whereas the term FTLD is used to indicate the neuropathology.

Thus, although from the 1980s through the early 2000s this approach was the traditional cutting edge of clinical practice in the diagnosis of patients with cognitive impairment, there has been a pressing need for biomarkers of underlying neuropathology.[3] As there are attempts to move toward developing therapies targeting specific molecular neurodegenerative pathologies, it has become clear that molecular biomarkers for inclusion and outcome measures are needed. Attention has been increasingly called to this issue as data accumulate demonstrating that there is no simple one-to-one relationship between a clinical phenotype and the specific pathology. For example, although a majority of patients with AD with amyloid plaques and neurofibrillary tangle pathology[4] present with the classic progressive episodic memory impairment, 5% of those above age 65

and up to a third of those below age 65 present with an atypical phenotype, which can include frontal variant, posterior cortical atrophy (PCA), the logopenic variant of PPA (lvPPA), and corticobasal syndrome (CBS).[5–8] Conversely, a well-defined clinical syndrome can have several possible underlying neuropathologies. For example, the diagnosis of CBS during life is notoriously inaccurate in predicting corticobasal degeneration (CBD) pathology, because patients with CBS may turn out to have tau-CBD, tau-PSP, tau-Pick disease, or AD pathology.[9] As for PPA, it is still challenging to predict the pathology for the agrammatic or lvPPA subtypes.[10]

Amyloid PET, a specific marker of one of the core features of AD pathology—neuritic amyloid plaques—has revolutionized the field of AD since its introduction more than a decade ago.[11] The recently updated diagnostic criteria for AD dementia[12] explicitly incorporate molecular biomarkers of disease pathology: amyloid PET and cerebrospinal fluid (CSF) amyloid and tau. Individuals with MCI who have a positive amyloid PET scan are generally viewed as having prodromal AD and are at greater likelihood than those with a negative amyloid PET scan to progress within a few years to dementia. Clinical trials are now targeting prodromal AD patients and multiple studies have used amyloid PET imaging to demonstrate a reduction of brain amyloid levels in patients treated with anti-amyloid antibody therapy (discussed later).

In the past few years, a series of studies has also begun to demonstrate potential uses of an imaging biomarker specific to tau pathology, which holds enormous promise not only for AD but also for other forms of dementia with underlying tauopathy, such as FTD. Unfortunately, despite tremendous effort, there are still not robust leads for biomarkers of TDP-43 or α-synuclein. This article discusses the clinical utility and research applications of amyloid and tau PET imaging and how they are enhancing knowledge of the basic pathophysiologic processes underlying various dementias and accelerating efforts aiming to develop effective disease-modifying therapies.

AMYLOID PET IMAGING
Clinical Use of Amyloid PET Imaging in Patients with Cognitive Impairment

[11C]Pittsburgh compound B ([11C]PiB), the first PET radiotracer specifically binding amyloid beta (Aβ) plaques, was introduced in 2004.[11] [11C]PiB retention is specific for Aβ neuritic plaque pathology; it does not bind to other protein deposits that frequently co-occur with amyloid, such as neurofibrillary tangles or α-synuclein.[13] Numerous studies over the years have demonstrated its validity by showing it to be highly correlated with in vivo CSF Aβ42 as well as Aβ pathology in autopsy specimens.[14] Despite the many in vivo and postmortem validation studies in its favor, one major drawback of [11C]PiB is its very short half-life of 20 minutes, limiting its use to centers with an on-site cyclotron for radiotracer production. Subsequent efforts have led to the development of a family of fluorinated compounds with longer half-lives, including [18F]florbetapir, [18F]flutametamol, and [18F]florbetaben. [18F]florbetapir was the first of these tracers to be approved by the US Food and Drug Administration in 2012, with [18F]flutametamol and [18F]florbetaben approved in 2013 and 2014, respectively. These tracers were approved after studies demonstrated that clinical readers could reliably interpret the scans in patients with a range of cognitive impairment and that scan results were sensitive and specific predictors of the presence of neuritic plaques in a subset of patients who were followed to autopsy.

As more has been learned about amyloid PET imaging in the decade since its introduction, guidelines for its clinical applicability have been extensively discussed. The use of amyloid PET imaging is considered most appropriate when patients present with cognitive impairment that could be attributed to AD pathology but where the clinician is uncertain and the confirmation of presence or absence of amyloid would change diagnostic confidence.[15] In other words, in a 70-year-old patient presenting with progressive episodic memory impairment with executive dysfunction, hippocampal atrophy, and temporoparietal hypometabolism, amyloid PET is not particularly helpful because most clinicians consider this patient likely to have typical amnesic AD dementia, and, therefore, a positive amyloid PET scan would not significantly alter the already high diagnostic confidence. On the other hand, use of amyloid PET imaging is particularly relevant

for patients presenting with phenotypes such as PCA, CBS, or PPA, in which AD is one of several possible underlying pathologies,[16–18] and the results of an amyloid PET scan could substantially change diagnostic confidence. In the United States, although amyloid PET imaging is FDA approved, it is not yet reimbursed by payors, limiting access. A study was recently launched that enables dementia specialists to order amyloid PET scans for Medicare subscribers over the age of 65 who meet appropriate use criteria: Imaging Dementia — Evidence for Amyloid Scanning (www.ideas-study.org). The Centers for Medicare & Medicaid Services has authorized reimbursement of the cost of scans in patients who are enrolled in this study of the clinical utility of amyloid PET imaging.

The crucial role of amyloid PET imaging can be illustrated by the case of a right-handed woman who presented at age 65 with a 6-year history of progressive language difficulties. Her speech and language profile consisted of difficulty retrieving single words and repeating sentences and phonologic errors in confrontation naming and spontaneous speech but no single word comprehension, grammar, or motor speech impairment. Memory, executive function, and visuospatial function were relatively preserved, as was comportment. Hypometabolism on FDG-PET was seen in the left temporal lobe and to a lesser degree in the left frontal lobe, with sparing of the posterior cingulate cortex. A diagnosis of lvPPA was made. Although most cases of lvPPA have underlying AD pathology, confidence was lower in this patient due to mild agrammatism, frontal involvement, and sparing of posterior cingulate cortex, raising the question of FTLD pathology. The use of amyloid PET scan, which showed increased [11C]PiB uptake most pronounced and extensive in bilateral medial frontal cortices, confirmed the presence of abundant neuritic plaques (**Fig. 1**). CSF analysis demonstrated reduced

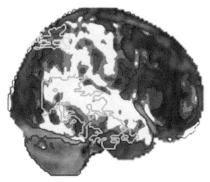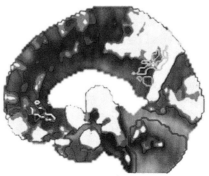

Fig. 1. Robustly elevated amyloid PET signal as measured with florbetapir PET in a patient with lvPPA viewed from the lateral surface (*left*) and medial surface (*right*).

Aβ and elevated phospho-tau. These molecular biomarkers strongly support the likely pathologic diagnosis of AD. Although measuring CSF amyloid is a potential alternative to amyloid PET imaging as a specific molecular biomarker for AD in clinical practice,[19] it is a more invasive procedure than PET imaging, which limits its use in many practice settings.

Amyloid PET Imaging in Preclinical Alzheimer Disease and Incidental Amyloidosis

Models of the pathophysiologic sequence of AD suggest that accumulation of Aβ occurs early in the neurodegenerative process. The plot of amyloid burden versus time is sigmoidal in shape, and the average duration from detectable levels of amyloid in vivo to levels where amyloid accumulates as plaques is estimated at approximately 15 to 20 years.[20] Numerous autopsy studies have shown that cognitively normal individuals followed prospectively to autopsy may have substantial amyloid plaque pathology,[21–23] especially so with increasing age.

One important implication of this observation is that it is likely that older individuals with cognitive impairment may have incidentally positive amyloid PET scans. That is, multiple pathologies in a patient with dementia become increasingly common with age. In some patients with multiple pathologies, plaques and tangles are less prominent than another neurodegenerative pathology and thus may be viewed as not likely a major contributor to symptoms.[4] The direct clinical implication is that, in a patient with cognitive impairment or dementia, a positive amyloid PET scan does not immediately indicate that AD is the underlying pathophysiologic process. A positive scan does not establish a diagnosis of AD. As with any test result, the clinician has to interpret an amyloid PET result in the context of the other information available. Discussions surrounding this issue were generated in part in relation to the presence of substantial brain amyloid in individuals who are cognitively normal.

It is important to recognize that it is not yet known whether, if they are followed for a long enough period of time, most or all amyloid-positive cognitively normal individuals go on to develop AD dementia. In cognitively normal older adults, there is a spectrum ranging from individuals harboring isolated cerebral amyloidosis with no evidence of neuronal injury (stage 1), to those with amyloid and neuronal injury (stage 2), to those with these 2 biomarkers as well as subtle symptoms of cognitive decline (not yet meeting criteria for MCI; stage 3).[24] This issue has recently been discussed as requiring a distinction between a cognitively normal older adult with evidence of both brain amyloid and brain tau—referred to as preclinical AD—as opposed to a cognitively normal older adult with evidence of only brain amyloid or brain tau—referred to asymptomatic at-risk for AD.[25]

Using Amyloid PET for Treatment Development

In addition to its clinical utility, amyloid PET imaging has revolutionized therapy development for AD. The use of amyloid PET scans as part of the inclusion criteria is now ensuring that patients enrolled in the trials have the pathophysiologic disease targeted by the therapy under study. Although these trials have so far produced disappointing results in terms of cognitive benefit, some have demonstrated a modest reduction in cerebral amyloidosis[26,27] and, recently, encouraging data were reported from a phase 1b study of the monoclonal antibody aducanumab.[28] After 1 year of monthly intravenous infusions of this drug, patients with prodromal or mild AD exhibited dose-dependent reductions in brain amyloid, accompanied by preliminary evidence of clinical benefit from the Clinical Dementia Rating scale and the Mini-Mental State Examination. A phase 3 trial is now in progress.

Amyloid PET Imaging in Other Dementias

Dementia with Lewy bodies and Parkinson disease with dementia

Aβ plaques, a hallmark pathology of AD, are also commonly observed in DLB and Parkinson disease with dementia (PDD).[29,30] Results of PET imaging studies using amyloid radiotracers agree with neuropathologic studies. DLB patients often have high levels of amyloid deposition compared with healthy controls.[31] Although fewer PDD patients have significant Aβ accumulation, some of them may still demonstrate levels of amyloid deposition in the AD range.[13] Higher amyloid deposition in DLB patients has been associated with greater cognitive impairment[32] and better response to cholinesterase inhibitors.[33] Higher amyloid deposition in Parkinson disease (PD) patients portends faster progression to dementia.[34] In addition to these associations with clinical outcomes, high cortical amyloid deposition has been shown to predict greater cortical and medial temporal lobe atrophy, anatomic changes classically associated with AD pathology.[35] Taken together, these findings suggest that the amyloidosis seen in DLB and PDD is not merely incidental but signifies that α-synucleinopathy may coexist with AD pathology. Even when the presence of amyloidosis does not meet criteria for a pathologic diagnosis of AD, PD patients with amyloidosis transition faster to dementia.[36] This persistent relationship between the severity of amyloid burden measured via PET imaging and cognitive impairment in PD and DLB suggests that the cognitive decline in these patients may be precipitated by a synergy between amyloid and α-synuclein.

Frontotemporal dementia
Amyloid PET imaging is usually negative in patients with the clinical syndrome of FTD[13,37]; therefore, it can in theory be used to exclude AD when the suspected underlying pathology is FTLD, clinically manifesting as behavioral variant FTD (bvFTD) or PPA. It is more complicated, however, in practice. When a patient clinically diagnosed with FTD has a positive amyloid scan, there are 3 possible explanations, as discussed previously: (1) the pathologic diagnosis is AD (eg, frontal variant AD[38]); (2) there is coexisting FTLD and AD (ie, mixed pathology) that both contribute to dementia; and (3) the amyloid in the patient is incidental with relatively low Braak-stage neurofibrillary degeneration and thus likely noncontributory to symptoms. Differentiating these possibilities may be possible with the clinical symptomatology itself and MR imaging or FDG-PET (eg, the prior probability that a patient with classical semantic variant PPA supported by MR imaging or FDG-PET has TDP-43 type C pathology is so high that a positive amyloid PET scan should be interpreted with caution). In many cases of suspected FTLD with a positive amyloid PET scan, however, an examination of CSF tau or tau PET may be helpful, which is discussed.

TAU PET IMAGING
Clinical Use of Tau PET Tracers in Alzheimer Disease

Although amyloid PET imaging has contributed tremendously to increasing diagnostic confidence in dementia patient evaluation, neuropathologic studies have long shown that the localization and magnitude of tau pathology correlate better than amyloid with neurodegeneration and clinical symptoms.[39] This has been confirmed with in vivo PET studies showing that the topography of amyloid deposition does not relate to clinical symptoms, especially in atypical subtypes of AD (eg, PCA, CBS, lvPPA, and frontal variant).[40–43]

Motivated in part by these issues, substantial effort has been devoted to the development of radiotracers to measure tau-related neurodegeneration. Most of these efforts to date have started by

identifying compounds that bind to hyperphosphorylated paired helical filament (PHF) tau in AD tissue. In the past few years, 3 main chemical classes of tau PET tracers, quinolone derivatives, benzothiazole derivatives, and benzimidazole pyrimidines, were developed and shown to selectively bind to PHF tau pathology.[44] Recently, an additional 3-pyrrolo[2,3]pyridine compound has also shown promise in an in vitro study.[45] **Table 1** lists the individual radiotracers in each chemical class.

Tau PET imaging in Alzheimer disease
Of the tracers available to date, [^{18}F]AV-1451 (previously known as [^{18}F]T807) has generated the most published data. The first in vivo images of [^{18}F]AV-1451 showed the expected uptake in temporal and parietal regions in patients with AD dementia and amnesic MCI likely of AD pathology.[46] Subsequently, it was also shown in larger samples that the topographic distribution of [^{18}F]AV-1451 in amnesic MCI or AD dementia, compared with normal aging, was consistent with Braak staging, with more prominent tracer binding in inferior and lateral temporoparietal cortices, parieto-occipital cortices, posterior cingulate cortices, and precuneus and less in frontal regions and primary sensorimotor cortices.[47,48] Similar results have been observed in AD dementia patients using other tau PET tracers, including [^{18}F]THK5351[49] and [^{11}C]PBB3.[50]

As predicted by previous postmortem studies, tau pathology as indexed by [^{18}F]AV-1451 binding also better correlated with severity and type of clinical symptoms than amyloid pathology. In typical amnesic AD dementia, [^{18}F]AV-1451 binding in inferior temporal gyrus correlated better with clinical impairment than [^{11}C]PiB.[47] The

Table 1
Tau radiotracers

Chemical Class	Radiotracer
Quinolone derivatives	[^{18}F]THK523 [^{18}F]THK5117 [^{18}F]THK5105 [^{18}F]THK5351
Benzothiazole derivatives	[^{11}C]PBB3
Benzimidazole pyrimidines	[^{18}F]AV-1451 or flortaucipir (previously known as [^{18}F]T807) [^{18}F]T808
3-pyrrolo[2,3] pyridine	[^{18}F]MK-6240

topography of tau PET signal differentiated between atypical AD phenotypes, such as PCA, CBS, lvPPA, and behavioral/dysexecutive phenotypes, with each demonstrating a distinct topography of [^{18}F]AV-1451 binding.[51,52] The authors have made similar observations (**Fig. 2**).[53]

Ossenkoppele and colleagues[51,54] also found that, in patients with atypical AD subtypes, compared with [^{11}C]PiB, topography of [^{18}F]AV-1451 binding colocalized better with hypometabolism measured via FDG-PET, and the degree of tracer binding correlated better with the severity of hypometabolism. The authors corroborated this finding, showing that [^{18}F]AV-1451 topography and severity colocalized and correlated better with cortical atrophy than [^{11}C]PiB in patients with atypical subtypes of AD.[53] Based on these and other observations, not only will tau PET likely be a critical additional clinical tool in diagnosing atypical subtypes of AD with more confidence but also it will complement amyloid imaging because it colocalizes with neurodegenerative lesions predictive of clinical symptoms much better than amyloid PET imaging.

Tau PET Imaging in Frontotemporal Dementia

Tau PET also presents opportunities to improve clinical care and research for the spectrum of disorders encompassed by FTLD pathologies, which includes primary tauopathies (Pick disease, PSP, and CBD) as well as TDP-43 proteinopathies. Although some patients with FTD have autosomal-dominant genetic mutations that allow the likely pathology to be inferred, most patients with FTD have a sporadic condition, which presents important challenges in considering the possible molecular pathology. For example, bvFTD is just as likely to result from tau pathology (eg, classic Pick disease) as it is from TDP-43 pathology. Thus, an obvious and critically important goal is to determine whether tau PET imaging is useful in identifying sporadic bvFTD patients who are tau-positive versus those who are tau-negative.

For the most part, however, the radioligands developed to date have been screened against PHF-tau in AD tissue. Tau deposits in non-AD tauopathies differ in biochemical and conformational properties; radiotracers that bind to the PHF-tau found in AD may not bind as avidly to straight filaments found in PSP and CBD or to twisted filaments found in Pick disease.[44] Initial postmortem studies demonstrate minimal or no binding of [^{18}F]AV1451 to non-AD tauopathies,[55,56] suggesting that current tracers will not likely generalize to FTLD. Preliminary in vivo studies, however, have also shown [^{18}F]AV-1451 to have increased uptake in frontal and temporal cortices of patients with FTLD, a pattern expected for distribution of tauopathy in FTLD.[57,58] Investigators are actively pursuing questions regarding why elevated signal has been seen in vivo but minimally or not at all in postmortem autoradiographic analyses and why elevated signal has been observed in vivo in some patients highly likely not to have a primary FTLD tauopathy (eg, semantic variant PPA). Other tracers, including [^{18}F] THK5351, are being investigated in the FTLD spectrum as well.

Tau PET Imaging in Lewy Body Disorders

Tau PET radiotracers can also be of value in DLB and PD, in which an AD-like tauopathy frequently coexists with the primary α-syncleinopathy. One recent study examining cortical tau deposition in cognitively impaired patients with PD and DLB showed that they do have increased in vivo cortical tau accumulation compared with healthy controls as measured by [^{18}F]AV-1451.[59] Although the levels of tau radiotracer binding were lower than that seen in AD patients, the topographic distribution of tau was similar to that seen in AD. In addition, the degree of cortical tau binding in the inferior temporal gyrus and precuneus, areas known to be particularly affected in AD, correlated with severity of cognitive impairment as measured by the Mini-Mental State Examination and Clinical Dementia Rating. This is in agreement with what is

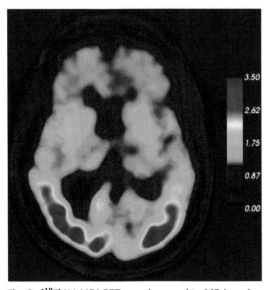

Fig. 2. [^{18}F]AV-1451 PET superimposed to MR imaging in a case of PCA with underlying Alzheimer dementia pathology; color bar displays legend for SUVR (standard uptake value ratios).

predicted from prior neuropathologic studies, which have shown a relationship between cortical tau deposition with cognitive impairment in Lewy body disease.[60] Even in some patients where PiB binding was low, higher than normal [^{18}F]AV-1451 deposition was detected, suggesting that amyloid and tau pathologies may occur through independent pathways in a subset of patients with Lewy body disease.

Primary Age-Related Tauopathy

Abnormal tau also occurs in clinically normal individuals, with its prevalence increasing dramatically with age. It can be detected in the medial and inferior temporal lobe (Braak stages I/II) in 10% of 20 year olds, 80% of 60 year olds, and 95% of 80 year olds, in the absence of amyloid pathology.[39,61] This pathologic entity has recently been named *primary age-related tauopathy*.[62] It is beginning to be studied in vivo, with some evidence that elevated tau PET signal can be seen in these brain regions in people who have biomarkers consistent with low amyloid.[47]

FUTURE DIRECTIONS

Although the pathogenesis of tau and Aβ pathologies are thought to be partially independent processes, some investigators hypothesize that the development of Aβ pathology accelerates the low-level tauopathy that may preexist, promoting the spread of tau pathology from subcortical or archicortical regions to isocortical areas, ultimately emerging as AD dementia.[63] Now that robust PET tracers are available for both pathologies, unprecedented experiments to better understand the independent and synergistic contributions of amyloid and tau in AD pathogenesis will be able to be performed. In addition, as efforts grow to develop therapeutic interventions aimed at tau pathology,[64–66] tau PET imaging will be a crucial biomarker to be used in these clinical trials.

Initial studies using tau PET have shown that, compared with amyloid pathology, tau pathology better predicts the localization and severity of neurodegeneration seen on structural MR imaging and FDG-PET. Future longitudinal studies using multimodal imaging may reveal the sequence and timing of how these events (ie, appearance of amyloid and tau pathology, change in metabolism, and reduction in cortical volume) unfold over the course of the neurodegenerative process. Eventually, combining tau PET imaging with functional MR imaging and diffusion tensor imaging may allow hypotheses to be tested about how hyperphosphorylated tau pathology relates to and may spread through the complex network architecture of the brain. The use of amyloid and tau PET in conjunction with functional brain imaging in cognitively normal individuals will help illuminate the processes present in the earliest preclinical phases of AD and related disorders. Finally, tau PET imaging will also likely contribute in important ways to clinical assessment of patients with disorders of cognition. The arsenal of weapons to fight these devastating diseases has never been stronger.

REFERENCES

1. Gorno-Tempini ML, Hillis A, Weintraub S, et al. Classification of primary progressive aphasia and its variants. Neurology 2011;76(11):1006–14.
2. Rascovsky K, Hodges JR, Knopman D, et al. Sensitivity of revised diagnostic criteria for the behavioural variant of frontotemporal dementia. Brain 2011; 134(Pt 9):2456–77.
3. Dickerson BC, Sperling RA. Neuroimaging biomarkers for clinical trials of disease-modifying therapies in Alzheimer's disease. NeuroRx 2005;2(2): 348–60.
4. Hyman BT, Phelps CH, Beach TG, et al. National institute on aging-Alzheimer's association guidelines for the neuropathologic assessment of Alzheimer's disease: a practical approach. Acta Neuropathol 2012;123(1):1–11.
5. Balasa M, Gelpi E, Antonell A, et al. Clinical features and APOE genotype of pathologically proven early-onset Alzheimer disease. Neurology 2011;76(20): 1720–5.
6. Snowden JS, Stopford CL, Julien CL, et al. Cognitive phenotypes in Alzheimer's disease and genetic risk. Cortex 2007;43(7):835–45.
7. Koedam EL, Lauffer V, Van Der Vlies AE, et al. Early-versus late-onset Alzheimer's disease: more than age alone. J Alzheimers Dis 2010;19(4):1401–8.
8. Warren JD, Fletcher PD, Golden HL. The paradox of syndromic diversity in Alzheimer disease. Nat Rev Neurol 2012;8(8):451–64.
9. Boeve BF, Maraganore DM, Parisi JE, et al. Pathologic heterogeneity in clinically diagnosed corticobasal degeneration. Neurology 1999;53(4):795–800.
10. Grossman M. Primary progressive aphasia: clinico-pathological correlations. Nat Rev Neurol 2010; 6(2):88–97.
11. Klunk WE, Engler H, Nordberg A, et al. Imaging brain amyloid in Alzheimer's disease with Pittsburgh Compound-B. Ann Neurol 2004;55(3):306–19.
12. McKhann GM, Knopman DS, Chertkow H, et al. The diagnosis of dementia due to Alzheimer's disease: recommendations from the National Institute on Aging-Alzheimer's Association workgroups on diagnostic guidelines for Alzheimer's disease. Alzheimers Dement 2011;7(3):263–9.

13. Villemagne VL, Ong K, Mulligan RS, et al. Amyloid imaging with 18F-florbetaben in Alzheimer disease and other dementias. J Nucl Med 2011;52(8):1210–7.

14. Jack CR, Barrio JR, Kepe V. Cerebral amyloid PET imaging in Alzheimer's disease. Acta Neuropathol 2013;126(5):643–57.

15. Johnson KA, Minoshima S, Bohnen NI, et al. Appropriate use criteria for amyloid PET: a report of the amyloid imaging task force, the society of nuclear medicine and molecular imaging, and the Alzheimer's association. J Nucl Med 2013;54(3):476–90.

16. Renner JA, Burns JM, Hou CE, et al. Progressive posterior cortical dysfunction: a clinicopathologic series. Neurology 2004;63(7):1175–80.

17. Ling H, O'Sullivan SS, Holton JL, et al. Does corticobasal degeneration exist? A clinicopathological re-evaluation. Brain 2010;133(7):2045–57.

18. Mesulam M, Wicklund A, Johnson N, et al. Alzheimer and frontotemporal pathology in subsets of primary progressive aphasia. Ann Neurol 2008;63(6):709–19.

19. Tapiola T, Alafuzoff I, Herukka S-K, et al. Cerebrospinal fluid {beta}-amyloid 42 and tau proteins as biomarkers of Alzheimer-type pathologic changes in the brain. Arch Neurol 2009;66(3):382–9.

20. Jack CR, Knopman DS, Jagust WJ, et al. Tracking pathophysiological processes in Alzheimer's disease: an updated hypothetical model of dynamic biomarkers. Lancet Neurol 2013;12(2):207–16.

21. Price JL, McKeel DW, Buckles VD, et al. Neuropathology of nondemented aging: Presumptive evidence for preclinical Alzheimer disease. Neurobiol Aging 2009;30(7):1026–36.

22. Price JL, Davis PB, Morris JC, et al. The distribution of tangles, plaques and related inmunohistochemical markers in healthy aging and Alzheimer's disease. Neurobiol Aging 1991;12(4):295–312.

23. Price JL, Morris JC. Tangles and plaques in nondemented aging and "preclinical" alzheimer's disease. Ann Neurol 1999;45(3):358–68.

24. Sperling RA, Aisen PS, Beckett LA, et al. Toward defining the preclinical stages of Alzheimer's disease: Recommendations from the National Institute on Aging-Alzheimer's Association workgroups on diagnostic guidelines for Alzheimer's disease. Alzheimers Dement 2011;7(3):280–92.

25. Dubois B, Hampel H, Feldman HH, et al. Preclinical Alzheimer's disease: definition, natural history, and diagnostic criteria. Alzheimers Dement 2016;12:292–323.

26. Salloway S, Sperling R, Fox NC, et al. Two phase 3 trials of bapineuzumab in mild-to-moderate Alzheimer's disease. N Engl J Med 2014;370(4):322–33.

27. Rinne JO, Brooks DJ, Rossor MN, et al. 11C-PiB PET assessment of change in fibrillar amyloid-?? load in patients with Alzheimer's disease treated with bapineuzumab: a phase 2, double-blind, placebo-controlled, ascending-dose study. Lancet Neurol 2010;9(4):363–72.

28. Sevigny J, Chiao P, Bussière T, et al. The antibody aducanumab reduces Aβ plaques in Alzheimer's disease. Nature 2016;537(7618):50–6.

29. Horvath J, Herrmann FR, Burkhard PR, et al. Neuropathology of dementia in a large cohort of patients with Parkinson's disease. Parkinsonism Relat Disord 2013;19(10):864–8.

30. Colom-Cadena M, Gelpi E, Charif S, et al. Confluence of alpha-synuclein, tau, and beta-amyloid pathologies in dementia with Lewy bodies. J Neuropathol Exp Neurol 2013;72(12):1203–12.

31. Gomperts SN, Rentz DM, Moran E, et al. Imaging amyloid deposition in Lewy body diseases. Neurology 2008;71(12):903–10.

32. Gomperts SN, Locascio JJ, Marquie M, et al. Brain amyloid and cognition in Lewy body diseases. Mov Disord 2012;27(8):965–73.

33. Graff-Radford J, Boeve BF, Pedraza O, et al. Imaging and acetylcholinesterase inhibitor response in dementia with Lewy bodies. Brain 2012;135(8):2470–7.

34. Gomperts S, Locascio J, Rentz D, et al. Amyloid is linked to cognitive decline in patients with Parkinson disease without dementia. Neurology 2013;80(1):85–91.

35. Shimada H, Shinotoh H, Hirano S, et al. B-amyloid in lewy body disease is related to Alzheimer's disease-like atrophy. Mov Disord 2013;28(2):169–75.

36. Sabbagh MN, Adler CH, Lahti TJ, et al. Parkinson disease with dementia: comparing patients with and without Alzheimer pathology. Alzheimer Dis Assoc Disord 2009;23(3):295–7.

37. Engler H, Santillo AF, Wang SX, et al. In vivo amyloid imaging with PET in frontotemporal dementia. Eur J Nucl Med Mol Imaging 2008;35(1):100–6.

38. Johnson JK, Head E, Kim R, et al. Clinical and pathological evidence for a frontal variant of Alzheimer disease. Arch Neurol 1999;56(10):1233–9.

39. Nelson PT, Alafuzoff I, Bigio EH, et al. Correlation of Alzheimer disease neuropathologic changes with cognitive status: a review of the literature. J Neuropathol Exp Neurol 2012;71(5):362–81.

40. Lehmann M, Ghosh PM, Madison C, et al. Diverging patterns of amyloid deposition and hypometabolism in clinical variants of probable Alzheimer's disease. Brain 2013;136(3):844–58.

41. Wolk DA, Price JC, Madeira C, et al. Amyloid imaging in dementias with atypical presentation. Alzheimers Dement 2012;8(5):389–98.

42. Rabinovici GD, Jagust WJ, Furst AJ, et al. Aβ amyloid and glucose metabolism in three variants of primary progressive aphasia. Ann Neurol 2008;64(4):388–401.

43. Rosenbloom MH, Alkalay A, Agarwal N, et al. Distinct clinical and metabolic deficits in PCA and AD are not related to amyloid distribution. Neurology 2011;76(21):1789–96.

44. Villemagne VL, Fodero-Tavoletti MT, Masters CL, et al. Tau imaging: early progress and future directions. Lancet Neurol 2015;14(1):114–24.

45. Hostetler ED, Walji AM, Zeng Z, et al. Preclinical characterization of 18F-MK-6240, a promising positron emission tomography (PET) tracer for in vivo quantification of human neurofibrillary tangles (NFTs). J Nucl Med 2016;57:1599–607.

46. Chien DT, Bahri S, Szardenings AK, et al. Early clinical PET imaging results with the novel PHF-Tau Radioligand [F-18]-T807. J Alzheimers Dis 2013;34(2): 457–68.

47. Johnson KA, Schultz A, Betensky RA, et al. Tau positron emission tomographic imaging in aging and early Alzheimer disease. Ann Neurol 2016;79(1): 110–9.

48. Schöll M, Lockhart SN, Schonhaut DR, et al. PET imaging of tau deposition in the aging human brain. Neuron 2016;89(5):971–82.

49. Harada R, Okamura N, Furumoto S, et al. 18F-THK5351: a novel PET radiotracer for imaging neurofibrillary pathology in Alzheimer's disease. J Nucl Med 2015;57(2):1–43.

50. Maruyama M, Shimada H, Suhara T, et al. Imaging of tau pathology in a tauopathy mouse model and in Alzheimer patients compared to normal controls. Neuron 2013;79(6):1094–108.

51. Ossenkoppele R, Schonhaut DR, Schöll M, et al. Tau PET patterns mirror clinical and neuroanatomical variability in Alzheimer's disease. Brain 2016; 139(Pt 5):1551–67.

52. Ossenkoppele R, Schonhaut DR, Baker SL, et al. Tau, amyloid, and hypometabolism in a patient with posterior cortical atrophy. Ann Neurol 2015;77(2): 338–42.

53. Xia C, Makaretz SJ, Caso C, et al. Association of in vivo [18F]AV-1451 tau PET imaging results with cortical atrophy and symptoms in typical and atypical Alzheimer disease. JAMA Neurol 2017; Epub ahead of print.

54. Ossenkoppele R, Pijnenburg YA, Perry DC, et al. The behavioural/dysexecutive variant of Alzheimer's disease: clinical, neuroimaging and pathological features. Brain 2015;138:2732–49.

55. Marquié M, Normandin MD, Vanderburg CR, et al. Validating novel tau positron emission tomography tracer [F-18]-AV-1451 (T807) on postmortem brain tissue. Ann Neurol 2015;78(5):787–800.

56. Sander K, Lashley T, Gami P, et al. Characterization of tau positron emission tomography tracer [18F]AV-1451 binding to postmortem tissue in Alzheimer's disease, primary tauopathies, and other dementias. Alzheimers Dement 2016;12(11):1116–24.

57. Ghetti B, Oblak AL, Boeve BF, et al. Invited review: frontotemporal dementia caused by microtubule-associated protein tau gene (MAPT) mutations: a chameleon for neuropathology and neuroimaging. Neuropathol Appl Neurobiol 2015;41(1):24–46.

58. Dickerson B, Domoto-Reilly K, Daisy S, et al. Imaging tau pathology in vivo in Ftld: initial experience with [18F] T807 pet. Alzheimers Dement 2014; 10(Suppl 4):P115.

59. Gomperts SN, Locascio JJ, Makaretz SJ, et al. Tau positron emission tomographic imaging in lewy body diseases. JAMA Neurol 2016;2129:1–8.

60. Jellinger KA, Attems J. Prevalence and impact of vascular and Alzheimer pathologies in Lewy body disease. Acta Neuropathol 2008;115(4):427–36.

61. Arriagada PV, Marzloff K, Hyman BT. Distribution of Alzheimer-type pathologic changes in nondemented elderly individuals matches the pattern in Alzheimer's disease. Neurology 1992;42(9):1681–8.

62. Crary JF, Trojanowski JQ, Schneider JA, et al. Primary age-related tauopathy (PART): a common pathology associated with human aging. Acta Neuropathol 2014;128(6):755–66.

63. Musiek ES, Holtzman DM. Origins of Alzheimer's disease. Curr Opin Neurol 2012;25(6):715–20.

64. Giacobini E, Gold G. Alzheimer disease therapy–moving from amyloid-β to tau. Nat Rev Neurol 2013;9(12):677–86.

65. Selkoe DJ. The therapeutics of Alzheimer's disease: where we stand and where we are heading. Ann Neurol 2013;74(3):328–36.

66. Yoshiyama Y, Lee VMY, Trojanowski JQ. Therapeutic strategies for tau mediated neurodegeneration. J Neurol Neurosurg Psychiatry 2013;84(7):784–95.

Novel Phenotypes Detectable with PET in Mood Disorders

Elevated Monoamine Oxidase A and Translocator Protein Level

Jeffrey Meyer, MD, PhD, FRCP(C)[a,b,*]

KEYWORDS

- Monoamine oxidase A • Inflammation • Translocator protein • Major depressive disorder • PET
- Serotonin

KEY POINTS

- Monoamine oxidase A (MAO-A) is an important enzyme that metabolizes monoamines, generates oxidative stress, and influences apoptosis.
- Increased level of MAO-A occurs in affect-modulating brain regions in major depressive disorder and conditions/illnesses associated with major depressive disorder.
- The translocator protein 18 kDa (TSPO) is overexpressed when microglial activation, an important component of neuroinflammation, is present.
- Increased TSPO level occur in affect-modulating brain regions in major depressive disorder and common comorbid illnesses.

INTRODUCTION

Increasingly, it is recognized that complex psychiatric disorders are composed of combinations of phenotypes that, individually, are not specific to 1 disorder. This concept has extended to major depressive disorder (MDD) and the PET radioligand field has a special role to contribute to this direction because it may be applied to develop highly selective radioligands that indicate processes that contribute to the pathophysiology of the disease. The application of these ligands may indicate the specificity of the pathology to MDD, the state dependence of the abnormality, its relationship to predisposition to disease onset, and its responsiveness to currently available treatments. These issues are pivotal in MDD, which is recognized as the leading cause of death and disability in moderate-income to high-income nations,[1] largely because of the high lifetime prevalence of 10% to 15%, and

Disclosure: Dr Meyer has received operating grant funds for other studies from Janssen, Bristol-Myers Squibb, Eli Lilly and Company, GlaxoSmithKline, Lundbeck, and SK Life Sciences in the past 5 years. Dr Meyer has been a consultant to Mylan, Lundbeck, Takeda, Teva, and Trius in the past 5 years. None of these companies participated in the design or execution of this study or in the writing of the manuscript. No other disclosures were reported. Dr Meyer is an inventor on three patents of blood markers to predict brain inflammation and/or to diagnose affective disorders and a dietary supplement to reduce depressed mood in postpartum. Dr Meyer is arranging collaborations with nutraceutical companies for the dietary supplement.

[a] Research Imaging Centre, Campbell Family Mental Health Research Institute, Centre for Addiction and Mental Health, Toronto, Ontario, Canada; [b] Department of Psychiatry, University of Toronto, 250 College Street, Toronto, Ontario M5T1R8, Canada
* Corresponding author. Department of Psychiatry, University of Toronto, 250 College Street, Toronto, Ontario M5T1R8, Canada.
E-mail address: jeffhughmeyer@yahoo.ca

PET Clin 12 (2017) 361–371
http://dx.doi.org/10.1016/j.cpet.2017.02.008
1556-8598/17/© 2017 Elsevier Inc. All rights reserved.

treatment resistance, which occurs in 50% of cases.[2,3] By identifying phenotypes with selective radioligands, PET is enabling a transition from a 1 pathology, 1 disease perspective to a viewpoint of combinations of multiple pathologies. It is anticipated that targeting individual pathologies may improve treatment response and prevent onset and/or progression of this illness. This article focuses on 2 markers in this context: increased monoamine oxidase A (MAO-A) level and increased level of neuroinflammatory marker translocator protein 18 kDa (TSPO) in regions implicated in affect regulation.

MONOAMINE OXIDASE A

MAO-A is an important enzyme located on the outer mitochondrial membranes of neurons and glia.[4] In human brain, MAO-A density is highest in locus coeruleus but it is also high in the cortex, hippocampus, and striatum; lower in cerebellar cortex; and very low in white matter.[4,5] MAO-A has several functions with direct relationships to generating depressed mood, such as metabolizing serotonin, norepinephrine, and dopamine because depletion of these neurochemicals, whether through precursor-depleting diets or medications that disrupt the synthesis or storage of these monoamines, is associated with depressed mood.[6] MAO-A is also important in neurodegeneration, because of its role in generating oxidative stress through the production of hydrogen peroxide and in predisposing to intrinsic apoptosis.[7–10]

Several PET radioligands have been developed for imaging MAO-A. Originally [11C]clorgyline was the only radioligand available, which had poor reversibility[11] but otherwise good qualities, and then subsequent advances led to highly reversible compounds of overall outstanding quality being able to provide an index of MAO-A binding in the gray matter where MAO-A density is mainly present (Table 1). The parameters reflecting total MAO-A from these methods tend to be highly correlated with the known MAO-A density.[23] The binding site of harmine to MAO-A has been identified as being in the center of the functional pocket of the MAO-A enzyme.[24] For PET centers without an on-site cyclotron, there is a lack of availability of a fully developed fluorinated radiotracer, a need likely to be met with the promising development of [18F]fluoroethylharmol.[14,17]

An asset of in vivo imaging is the ease with which samples may be selectively chosen, which has been key for investigations of MAO-A in MDD. The MAO-A target was initially overlooked as a pathophysiologic marker of MDD, because the first postmortem study of MAO-A activity evaluated cases of suicide and the second had considerable focus on late-onset MDD.

Because only 50% of people who commit suicide have MDD,[25] and inheriting low MAO-A level may also be associated with neurodevelopment of pathologic impulsivity,[26] which is another component of risk for suicide, this study cannot be viewed as definitive for the issue of whether there is an alteration of MAO-A level or activity in MDD. Late-onset MDD is often associated with the neuropathologically different illnesses of Parkinson's disease and Alzheimer's disease.[27] In contrast, the most common, early-onset MDD, is associated with stressful events in its onset and evidence has gradually accumulated showing that chronic glucocorticoids increase transcription, level, and activity of MAO-A through direct binding to the promotor and influencing nuclear transcription factors.[28]

The first definitive study of MAO-A in early onset MDD applied [11C] harmine PET, and MAO-A V_S, an index of MAO-A density, was measured in medication-free major depressive episodes (MDE).[29] The MAO-A V_S was highly significantly increased (P<.001 each region, average magnitude 34% [or 2 standard deviations]) during MDE (Fig. 1). The sample of this study was focused on the effect of diagnosis of early-onset MDD, excluding psychiatric and medical comorbidity, to focus on the diagnostic difference. Subjects with MDE were drug free for at least 5 months and most were antidepressant naive. Additional consistent findings have emerged across diverse methods: Barton and colleagues[30] reported a consistent finding of increased brain serotonin turnover in unmedicated depressed patients. Also, the finding of greater MAO-A binding in MDE was replicated with [11C] harmine PET.[31] In 2011 the finding was replicated in antidepressant-free MDE subjects in a postmortem study of orbitofrontal cortex applying Western blot[7] and a similar increase in MAO-A activity was found. R1 is a nuclear transcription factor that inhibits MAO-A synthesis and, at reduced level, is implicated in apoptosis. R1 level is reduced in the prefrontal cortex (PFC) in MDD and its reduction correlates with the increase of MAO-A density.[7] Transforming growth factor beta-inducible early gene 2 (TIEG2) is a nuclear transcription factor that regulates genes participating in apoptosis and promotes MAO-A synthesis. TIEG2 level is increased in the PFC in MDD, and its increase correlates with the increase of MAO-A density in MDD.[8,32] The replication finding of [11C]harmine PET was extended to 42 patients with MDE and 37 healthy controls, showing the greatest level of MAO-A in those with greater severity and/or reversed neurovegetative symptoms (hypersomnia, hyperphagia, or weight gain).[33]

With regard to phase of illness, increased MAO-A level is persistent in MDD beyond the MDE, particularly in the PFC and anterior cingulate

Table 1
Comparison of PET radiotracers for monoamine oxidase A[34]

	[11C]Clorgyline	[11C]Harmine	[11C]Befloxatone	[18F]Fluoroethylharmol
Selectivity	Excellent[11]	Excellent[12]	Excellent[13]	Excellent[14]
Reversibility	Not reversible[11]	Highly reversible[15]	Highly reversible[16]	Moderate in rodent[14,17]
Brain Uptake	Very good[11]	High[15]	High[18]	Very good[14,17]
Modeling	2-tissue compartment[11]	2-tissue compartment[15]	2-tissue compartment[18]	Not yet completed in humans
Specific Binding to Free and Nonspecific Binding Ratio	Very good but limited assessment[11]	High ~4[15,19]	High in baboon[16]	High in rodent[14,17]
Reliability in Humans	Very good[20]	Excellent[21]	Not reported	Not yet completed
Brain Penetrant Radioactive Metabolites?	Unlikely	No brain penetrant metabolites[22]	Unlikely	No brain penetrant metabolites[17]
Can Be Measured in Diverse Regions?	Gray matter[11]	Gray matter[15]	Gray matter[18]	Gray matter in rodent[14,17]

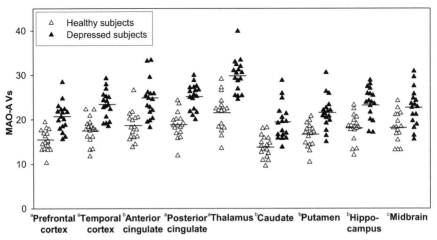

Fig. 1. Greater MAO-A–specific distribution volumes (V_s) during MDEs. On average, MAO-A V_s (index of specific binding of [^{11}C]harmine) was increased by 34%, or 2 standard deviations in MDE. Differences between groups were highly significant in each region. Significance of analyses of variance results: [a] $P = .00001$, [b] $P = .0001$, [c] $P = .001$. (*From* Meyer JH, Ginovart N, Boovariwala A, et al. Elevated monoamine oxidase A level in the brain: an explanation for the monoamine imbalance of major depression. Arch Gen Psychiatry 2006;63(11):1212; with permission.)

cortex (ACC), remaining increased beyond selective serotonin reuptake inhibitor (SSRI) treatment in both within-subject studies with [^{11}C]harmine PET imaging of MAO-A distribution volume (V_T), and the between-subject design of postmortem studies with Western blot.[7,31] When MAO-A V_T is increased in the PFC and ACC during recovery, it is associated with recurrence,[31] which characterizes an important facet of the monoamine theory of MDD: increased MAO-A V_T may be considered an index of a monoamine level–lowering process and, in the 1950s during treatment with reserpine-based antihypertensives, chronic monoamine level lowering was associated with subsequent onset of MDEs, which typically occurred 2 weeks to 4 months later.[35] Hence increased MAO-A level, particularly in the PFC and ACC, can be viewed as a common pathologic phenotype that persists through common SSRI treatments, and is implicated in recurrent MDE.

Increased MAO-A V_T, measured with [^{11}C]harmine PET, particularly in the PFC and ACC, is present in several illnesses associated with depressed mood and in high-risk states for MDE. These illnesses include early withdrawal from alcohol dependence, early withdrawal from heavy cigarette smoking, and borderline personality disorder.[36–38] Mechanistically, the most plausible reasons for the first 2 phenomena are that MAO-A level and activity increase after exposure to neurotoxins,[39] whereas exposure to high stress during development and in adulthood may account for increased MAO-A level in borderline personality disorder (as previously mentioned,

glucocorticoids bind to the MAO-A promotor and promote production of nuclear transcription factors[28]). Although all of these conditions are highly comorbid with MDE, and predispose to MDE, there are other conditions that frequently precede MDE. Examples include early postpartum and perimenopause, which are associated with increased MAO-A level across gray matter regions of 43% and 34% respectively[40,41] (**Fig. 2** shows a voxel-based display of the differential increase of MAO-A V_T in early postpartum). Postpartum MDE has a 13% prevalence and new-onset MDE in perimenopause has a 17% prevalence; strongly increased MAO-A V_T,[42,43] which occurs in both states, is the most prominent biological change common to MDE and these high-risk states for MDE. These findings indicate intriguing potential for novel prevention strategies to target increased MAO-A level or sequelae of increased MAO-A level, which is an essential issue because there are no standard approaches for preventing MDE onset in postpartum or perimenopause.

Inhibitors of MAO-A have been applied as antidepressants since their serendipitous discovery through past treatments for tuberculosis, in which some medications both inhibited MAO-A and reversed depressive symptoms. Occupancy data are now available for the irreversible inhibitor phenelzine, which potently reduces MAO-A V_T by 82% to 93% at clinical doses.[19] Moclobemide, a newer MAO-A inhibitor with a superior tolerability profile, has a lower occupancy at standard treating doses and can only reduce MAO-A V_T to a similar extend if the dosage is increased beyond the usual

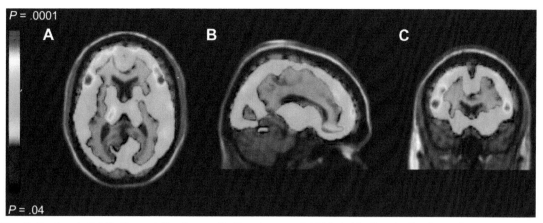

Fig. 2. Regional distribution of *P* values reflecting increased MAO-A binding in the immediate postpartum period. Parametric maps of increased MAO-A binding in the postpartum group versus the control group. Individual voxel threshold was set at *P*<.05; 86,412 voxels comprised a single cluster, which had a cluster-corrected significance of *P* = .03. Mean regional difference was 43% (*A–C* represent transverse, sagittal, and coronal views). (*From* Sacher J, Wilson A, Houle S, et al. Elevated brain monoamine oxidase A binding in early postpartum. Arch Gen Psychiatry 2010;67(5):471; with permission.)

directed daily dose.[19,44] The magnitude of inhibition associated with therapeutic effect in clinical trials exceeds the level of disease effect. However, there are several potential reasons for this, namely that the disease effect is persistent for months to years before treatment and it may be that downstream consequences of chronically increased MAO-A level are more likely to ameliorate after a greater degree of reversal. Moreover, it is also known that some antidepressant mechanisms, such as inducing signal transduction effects and inducing hippocampal neurogenesis, are associated with treatments that increase monoamine level beyond healthy state.[44]

TRANSLOCATOR PROTEIN IMAGING

Microglia represent 5% to 15% of brain cells and have an important monitoring role for the immune surveillance system, in which they detect inflammatory signals such as damage-associated molecular patterns, pathogen-associated molecular patterns, and cytokines.[42] In response to such stimuli, microglia become activated, and change their morphology to shift function from a detection state to a response state.[42,43] In this transformation, their dendrites change from being longer and more slender dendrites to being thickened with shorter and fewer dendrites, having a larger cell body volume, and sometimes becoming ameboid.[45,46] When microglia become activated, they overexpress TSPO, hence TSPO binding represents an important marker of neuroinflammation.[47] Although there has been some discussion regarding whether increased TSPO level may represent activated

microglia versus astroglia, empirically, after exposure to stroke, toxins, and lipopolysaccharide administration, the temporal magnitude of the increase in TSPO level closely matches markers associated with microglial activation but not markers associated with astroglial activation.[48–50]

In the early 1990s the only PET radioligand for translocator protein was [11C](*R*)-PK11195. Formal modeling quantification was delayed in humans until 2006, which showed much better properties for applying this radiotracer with a 2-tissue compartment and arterial sampling versus reference tissue approaches, presumably because no brain region with free and nondisplaceable binding characteristics representative of gray matter have been shown to be substantially devoid of TSPO receptors. A new generation of TSPO-binding radiotracers emerged over the mid to late 2000s that show greatly improved specific binding to free and nondisplaceable binding characteristics. There are several such radiotracers and a representative sample includes [11C]PBR28, [18F]FEPPA, [18F]PBR111, and [11C]ER176 (**Table 2**). [11C]PBR28 is probably the most widely applied technique but [18F]FEPPA is also applied at several sites. They are similar, although [11C]PBR28 has slightly less stable V_T values over the PET scanning period in humans and there are some (but not completely consistent) reports of radioactive, brain-penetrant metabolites in rodent brain.[52,53] The design of [18F]PBR111 sacrifices some of its ratio of specific binding to free and nondisplaceable binding for excellent reversibility of its time-activity curve, which is an asset for white matter imaging. It has fewer quantifiable regions because of

366 Meyer

Table 2
Comparison of PET radiotracers for translocator protein 18 kDa

	[11C](R)-PK11195	[11C]PBR28	[18F]FEPPA	[18F]PBR111	[11C]ER176
Selectivity	High[51]	High[52]	Excellent[53]	High[54]	Yes[55]
Reversibility	Very good[56]	Very good[57]	Good in gray matter[58]	Excellent[59]	Yes[60]
Brain Uptake	Good[61]	Very good[57]	Excellent[58]	Very good[59]	Very good[60]
Modeling	2-tissue compartment[56]	2-tissue compartment[57]	2-tissue compartment[58]	2-tissue compartment[59]	2-tissue compartment[60]
Specific Binding to Free and Nonspecific Binding Ratio	Modest with arterial sampling Low with reference tissue[56]	Very good[57]	High[58]	Very good[59]	Very good[60]
Reliability	Good for whole brain; poor for regions[61]	Yes in gray matter[62]	Good (personal communication)	Not yet published	Not yet published
Brain Penetrant Radioactive Metabolites?	Unlikely[63]	Negligible to low[52,53]	Less than minimum of quantitation[53]	Negligible[54]	Not yet published
Can Be Measured in Diverse Regions	Reliability best for whole brain regions[61]	Yes	Yes	Yes[60]	Yes

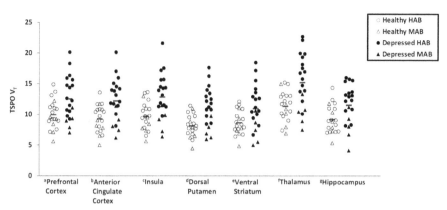

Fig. 3. Increased TSPO density (TSPO V_T) during an MDE secondary to MDD. TSPO V_T was significantly greater in MDE of MDD (depressed, N = 20, 15 high-affinity binders [HAB], 5 mixed-affinity binders [MAB]) compared with controls (healthy, N = 20, 14 HAB, 6 MAB). All second-generation TSPO radioligands, such as [^{18}F]FEPPA, show differential binding according to the single nucleotide polymorphism rs6971 of the TSPO gene resulting in HAB and MAB. Red bars indicate means in each group. Analysis of variance results are: [a] PFC, $F_{1,37}$ = 8.07, P = .007; [b] ACC, $F_{1,37}$ = 12.24, P = .001; [c] insula, $F_{1,37}$ = 12.34, P = .001; [d] dorsal putamen, $F_{1,37}$ = 14.1, P = .001; [e] ventral striatum, $F_{1,37}$ = 6.9, P = .013; [f] thalamus, $F_{1,37}$ = 13.6, P = .001; [g] hippocampus, $F_{1,37}$ = 7.5, P = .009. (*From* Setiawan E, Wilson AA, Mizrahi R, et al. Role of translocator protein density, a marker of neuroinflammation, in the brain during major depressive episodes. JAMA Psychiatry 2015;72(3):271; with permission.)

binding of radioactive metabolite to bone. [^{11}C] ER176 is at an earlier stage of development because it is newer. It is interesting insofar as its V_T measure is much less affected by the homozygous state of single nucleotide polymorphism rs6971,[59] found in 1% to 10% of patients, depending on their ethnicity (for other second-generation radioligands, patients who are homozygous for this genotype are typically excluded from applied neuroimaging studies). This polymorphism causes a single amino acid substitution that reduces the binding of TSPO to all second-generation radioligands. Although reliability of TSPO V_T for most ligands has not been formally reported, it is common for such data to remain unpublished during the first several years of radiotracer application.

TSPO PET imaging has been applied to discover that microglial activation occurs during MDE. In an [^{18}F]FEPPA PET study of 20 unmedicated patients with MDE with no active comorbid psychiatric illnesses and 20 controls the TSPO-specific V_T, an index of TSPO density, was significantly increased in the primary regions of the PFC, ACC, and insular cortex by a substantial magnitude of 30%[64] (**Fig. 3**). Although the finding was evident in the a priori selected regions, TSPO V_T was also increased throughout the other gray matter regions sampled. Consistent with this finding, Innis and colleagues[65] reported greater TSPO V_T within the gray matter regions assessed, including subregions of the PFC and ACC, in 11 unmedicated MDE subjects.

Although an [^{11}C]PBR28 PET study found no difference between patients and controls across a range of gray matter regions in a sample of 10 subjects with MDD,[50] only half were in the midst of a current MDE. Earlier postmortem investigations of microglial activation in gray matter, which, although not focused on MDD in terms of sample size, tended to have consistent results, with positive findings being more likely in those sampling current MDE and negative findings being more likely in samples not selecting current MDE. In a study of individuals who committed suicide, who are more likely to have current psychiatric illness, Steiner and colleagues[66] reported increased density of cells positive for quinolinic acid, a marker influenced by microglial activation, in the ACC of 7 subjects with MDE. Another study in suicides reported greater staining with human leukocyte antigen-antigen D related (HLA-DR), a marker of microglial activation, in the dorsolateral PFC and ACC and it included 9 subjects with MDD.[67] In a sample less oriented toward current MDE, Van Otterloo and colleagues[68] reported no difference in density of activated microglia in the white matter of the orbitofrontal region in 10 subjects with MDD.

Parameters of increased TSPO binding throughout gray matter are not specific to MDD, being also found in Alzheimer disease[69,70] and concussion[71]; however, these other disorders are associated with a high prevalence of comorbid MDD. Microglial activation can be a nonselective response to many different cerebral insults, but, in contrast with these other diseases, for which it is less evident that the cardinal symptoms are induced by inflammation or microglial activation, induction of inflammation by cytokines, vaccines, and lipopolysaccharide is associated with the depressed mood and behaviors of MDD.[64]

SUMMARY AND FUTURE DIRECTIONS

A particular challenge for investigations of MDD is its heterogeneity, and both MAO-A and TSPO PET imaging show great promise in discerning phenotypes associated with MDE. The quality of radioligands for MAO-A and TSPO each had significant advances after the initial compounds. For MAO-A, later compounds show more reversibility and, for TSPO, the ratio of specific to free and nonspecific binding was considerably increased in the radioligands developed after [^{11}C](R)-PK11195. It is interesting that the phenotype match to MDD is not fully selective for either increased MAO-A binding or increased TSPO binding in affect-modulating brain regions because such changes also occur in diseases and conditions associated with high rates of MDE symptoms and MDD itself. The application of PET has also enabled quantitation of MAO-A inhibitor effects on its binding in vivo, but the optimal translation to MDD still requires further development of low-cost predictors for the high–MAO-A phenotype coupled with broadly usable MAO-A inhibitor therapeutics. It is anticipated that future MAO-A inhibitors will have fewer incompatibilities with other medications, and, at doses associated with MAO-A occupancies in the 80% to 85% range, should result in higher rates of therapeutic response. For TSPO imaging, ongoing priorities include developing low-cost predictors of the increased TPSO V_T phenotype, and assessing therapeutic effects on the TSPO V_T, for which TSPO PET imaging can play an important role, to ultimately assist in matching MDE cases with increased microglial activation to a therapeutic that reduces or modulates microglial activation.

REFERENCES

1. World Health Organization. The global burden of disease: 2004 update. Switzerland: Department of Health Statistics and Informatics, Information Evidence and Research Cluster, WHO; 2008.
2. Trivedi MH, Rush AJ, Wisniewski SR, et al. Evaluation of outcomes with citalopram for depression using measurement-based care in STAR*D: implications for clinical practice. Am J Psychiatry 2006;163(1):28–40.
3. Patten SB. Accumulation of major depressive episodes over time in a prospective study indicates that retrospectively assessed lifetime prevalence estimates are too low. BMC Psychiatry 2009;9:19.
4. Saura J, Bleuel Z, Ulrich J, et al. Molecular neuroanatomy of human monoamine oxidases A and B revealed by quantitative enzyme radioautography and in situ hybridization histochemistry. Neuroscience 1996;70(3):755–74.
5. Saura J, Kettler R, Da Prada M, et al. Quantitative enzyme radioautography with 3H-Ro 41-1049 and 3H-Ro 19-6327 in vitro: localization and abundance of MAO-A and MAO-B in rat CNS, peripheral organs, and human brain. J Neurosci 1992;12(5):1977–99.
6. Ruhe HG, Mason NS, Schene AH. Mood is indirectly related to serotonin, norepinephrine and dopamine levels in humans: a meta-analysis of monoamine depletion studies. Mol Psychiatry 2007;12(4):331–59.
7. Johnson S, Stockmeier CA, Meyer JH, et al. The reduction of R1, a novel repressor protein for monoamine oxidase A, in major depressive disorder. Neuropsychopharmacology 2011;36(10):2139–48.
8. Grunewald M, Johnson S, Lu D, et al. Mechanistic role for a novel glucocorticoid-KLF11 (TIEG2) protein pathway in stress-induced monoamine oxidase A expression. J Biol Chem 2012;287(29):24195–206.
9. Ou XM, Chen K, Shih JC. Monoamine oxidase A and repressor R1 are involved in apoptotic signaling pathway. Proc Natl Acad Sci U S A 2006;103(29):10923–8.
10. Youdim MB, Edmondson D, Tipton KF. The therapeutic potential of monoamine oxidase inhibitors. Nat Rev Neurosci 2006;7(4):295–309.
11. Fowler JS, MacGregor RR, Wolf AP, et al. Mapping human brain monoamine oxidase A and B with 11C-labeled suicide inactivators and PET. Science 1987;235(4787):481–5.
12. Bergstrom M, Westerberg G, Langstrom B. 11C-harmine as a tracer for monoamine oxidase A (MAO-A): in vitro and in vivo studies. Nucl Med Biol 1997;24(4):287–93.
13. Dolle F, Valette H, Bramoulle Y, et al. Synthesis and in vivo imaging properties of [11C]befloxatone: a novel highly potent positron emission tomography ligand for mono-amine oxidase-A. Bioorg Med Chem Lett 2003;13(10):1771–5.
14. Schieferstein H, Piel M, Beyerlein F, et al. Selective binding to monoamine oxidase A: in vitro and in vivo evaluation of (18)F-labeled beta-carboline derivatives. Bioorg Med Chem 2015;23(3):612–23.
15. Ginovart N, Meyer JH, Boovariwala A, et al. Positron emission tomography quantification of [11C]-harmine binding to monoamine oxidase-A in the human brain. J Cereb Blood Flow Metab 2006;26(3):330–44.
16. Bottlaender M, Valette H, Delforge J, et al. In vivo quantification of monoamine oxidase A in baboon brain: a PET study using [(11)C]befloxatone and the multi-injection approach. J Cereb Blood Flow Metab 2010;30(4):792–800.
17. Maschauer S, Haller A, Riss PJ, et al. Specific binding of [(18)F]fluoroethyl-harmol to monoamine

oxidase A in rat brain cryostat sections, and compartmental analysis of binding in living brain. J Neurochem 2015;135(5):908–17.

18. Zanotti-Fregonara P, Leroy C, Roumenov D, et al. Kinetic analysis of [11C]befloxatone in the human brain, a selective radioligand to image monoamine oxidase A. EJNMMI Res 2013;3(1):78.

19. Chiuccariello L, Cooke RG, Miler L, et al. Monoamine oxidase-A occupancy by moclobemide and phenelzine: implications for the development of monoamine oxidase inhibitors. Int J Neuropsychopharmacol 2016;19(1):1–9.

20. Fowler JS, Volkow ND, Wang GJ, et al. Brain monoamine oxidase A inhibition in cigarette smokers. Proc Natl Acad Sci U S A 1996;93(24):14065–9.

21. Sacher J, Rabiner EA, Clark M, et al. Dynamic, adaptive changes in MAO-A binding after alterations in substrate availability: an in vivo [(11)C]-harmine positron emission tomography study. J Cereb Blood Flow Metab 2012;32(3):443–6.

22. Wilson A, Meyer J, Garcia A, et al. Determination of the arterial input function of the MAO-A inhibitor [11C] harmine in human subjects [abstract]. J Labelled Compounds Radiopharm 2003;46(S1):S367.

23. Tong J, Meyer JH, Furukawa Y, et al. Distribution of monoamine oxidase proteins in human brain: implications for brain imaging studies. J Cereb Blood Flow Metab 2013;33(6):863–71.

24. Son SY, Ma J, Kondou Y, et al. Structure of human monoamine oxidase A at 2.2-A resolution: the control of opening the entry for substrates/inhibitors. Proc Natl Acad Sci U S A 2008;105(15):5739–44.

25. Barraclough B, Bunch J, Nelson B, et al. A hundred cases of suicide: clinical aspects. Br J Psychiatry 1974;125:355–73.

26. Kolla NJ, Matthews B, Wilson AA, et al. Lower monoamine oxidase-A total distribution volume in impulsive and violent male offenders with antisocial personality disorder and high psychopathic traits: an [(11)C] harmine positron emission tomography study. Neuropsychopharmacology 2015;40(11):2596–603.

27. Krishnan KR. Biological risk factors in late life depression. Biol Psychiatry 2002;52(3):185–92.

28. Ou XM, Chen K, Shih JC. Glucocorticoid and androgen activation of monoamine oxidase A is regulated differently by R1 and Sp1. J Biol Chem 2006;281(30):21512–25.

29. Meyer JH, Ginovart N, Boovariwala A, et al. Elevated monoamine oxidase a levels in the brain: an explanation for the monoamine imbalance of major depression. Arch Gen Psychiatry 2006;63(11):1209–16.

30. Barton DA, Esler MD, Dawood T, et al. Elevated brain serotonin turnover in patients with depression: effect of genotype and therapy. Arch Gen Psychiatry 2008;65(1):38–46.

31. Meyer JH, Wilson AA, Sagrati S, et al. Brain monoamine oxidase A binding in major depressive disorder: relationship to selective serotonin reuptake inhibitor treatment, recovery, and recurrence. Arch Gen Psychiatry 2009;66(12):1304–12.

32. Harris S, Johnson S, Duncan JW, et al. Evidence revealing deregulation of the KLF11-MAO A pathway in association with chronic stress and depressive disorders. Neuropsychopharmacology 2015;40(6):1373–82.

33. Chiuccariello L, Houle S, Miler L, et al. Elevated monoamine oxidase a binding during major depressive episodes is associated with greater severity and reversed neurovegetative symptoms. Neuropsychopharmacology 2014;39(4):973–80.

34. Meyer JH. Monoamine oxidase A and serotonin transporter imaging with positron emission tomography. In: Dierckx R, Otte A, de Vries EFJ, et al, editors. PET and SPECT of neurobiological systems. Springer; 2014. p. 711–39.

35. Freis ED. Mental depression in hypertensive patients treated for long periods with large doses of reserpine. N Engl J Med 1954;251(25):1006–8.

36. Bacher I, Houle S, Xu X, et al. Monoamine oxidase a binding in the prefrontal and anterior cingulate cortices during acute withdrawal from heavy cigarette smoking. Arch Gen Psychiatry 2011;68(8):817–26.

37. Matthews BA, Kish SJ, Xu X, et al. Greater monoamine oxidase a binding in alcohol dependence. Biol Psychiatry 2014;75(10):756–64.

38. Kolla NJ, Chiuccariello L, Wilson AA, et al. Elevated monoamine oxidase-A distribution volume in borderline personality disorder is associated with severity across mood symptoms, suicidality, and cognition. Biol Psychiatry 2016;79(2):117–26.

39. Fitzgerald JC, Ugun-Klusek A, Allen G, et al. Monoamine oxidase-A knockdown in human neuroblastoma cells reveals protection against mitochondrial toxins. FASEB J 2014;28(1):218–29.

40. Sacher J, Wilson A, Houle S, et al. Elevated brain monoamine oxidase A binding in early postpartum. Arch Gen Psychiatry 2010;67(5):468–74.

41. Rekkas PV, Wilson AA, Lee VW, et al. Greater monoamine oxidase a binding in perimenopausal age as measured with carbon 11-labeled harmine positron emission tomography. JAMA Psychiatry 2014;71(8):873–9.

42. Kreutzberg GW. Microglia: a sensor for pathological events in the CNS. Trends Neurosci 1996;19(8):312–8.

43. Gehrmann J, Matsumoto Y, Kreutzberg GW. Microglia: intrinsic immuneffector cell of the brain. Brain Res Brain Res Rev 1995;20(3):269–87.

44. Sacher J, Houle S, Parkes J, et al. Monoamine oxidase A inhibitor occupancy during treatment of major depressive episodes with moclobemide or St. John's wort: an [(11)C]-harmine PET study. J Psychiatry Neurosci 2011;36(6):375–82.

45. Carbonell WS, Murase S, Horwitz AF, et al. Migration of perilesional microglia after focal brain injury and

modulation by CC chemokine receptor 5: an in situ time-lapse confocal imaging study. J Neurosci 2005;25(30):7040–7.

46. Cross AK, Woodroofe MN. Chemokines induce migration and changes in actin polymerization in adult rat brain microglia and a human fetal microglial cell line in vitro. J Neurosci Res 1999;55(1):17–23.

47. Venneti S, Wiley CA, Kofler J. Imaging microglial activation during neuroinflammation and Alzheimer's disease. J Neuroimmune Pharmacol 2009;4(2):227–43.

48. Banati RB, Myers R, Kreutzberg GW. PK ('peripheral benzodiazepine')–binding sites in the CNS indicate early and discrete brain lesions: microautoradiographic detection of [3H]PK11195 binding to activated microglia. J Neurocytol 1997;26(2):77–82.

49. Martin A, Boisgard R, Theze B, et al. Evaluation of the PBR/TSPO radioligand [(18)F]DPA-714 in a rat model of focal cerebral ischemia. J Cereb Blood Flow Metab 2010;30(1):230–41.

50. Hannestad J, DellaGioia N, Gallezot JD, et al. The neuroinflammation marker translocator protein is not elevated in individuals with mild-to-moderate depression: a [(11)C]PBR28 PET study. Brain Behav Immun 2013;33:131–8.

51. Medran-Navarrete V, Damont A, Peyronneau MA, et al. Preparation and evaluation of novel pyrazolo [1,5-a]pyrimidine acetamides, closely related to DPA-714, as potent ligands for imaging the TSPO 18kDa with PET. Bioorg Med Chem Lett 2014; 24(6):1550–6.

52. Imaizumi M, Kim HJ, Zoghbi SS, et al. PET imaging with [11C]PBR28 can localize and quantify upregulated peripheral benzodiazepine receptors associated with cerebral ischemia in rat. Neurosci Lett 2007;411(3):200–5.

53. Wilson AA, Garcia A, Parkes J, et al. Radiosynthesis and initial evaluation of [18F]-FEPPA for PET imaging of peripheral benzodiazepine receptors. Nucl Med Biol 2008;35(3):305–14.

54. Fookes CJ, Pham TQ, Mattner F, et al. Synthesis and biological evaluation of substituted [18F] imidazo[1,2-a]pyridines and [18F]pyrazolo[1,5-a] pyrimidines for the study of the peripheral benzodiazepine receptor using positron emission tomography. J Med Chem 2008;51(13):3700–12.

55. Zanotti-Fregonara P, Zhang Y, Jenko KJ, et al. Synthesis and evaluation of translocator 18 kDa protein (TSPO) positron emission tomography (PET) radioligands with low binding sensitivity to human single nucleotide polymorphism rs6971. ACS Chem Neurosci 2014;5(10):963–71.

56. Kropholler MA, Boellaard R, Schuitemaker A, et al. Evaluation of reference tissue models for the analysis of [11C](R)-PK11195 studies. J Cereb Blood Flow Metab 2006;26(11):1431–41.

57. Fujita M, Imaizumi M, Zoghbi SS, et al. Kinetic analysis in healthy humans of a novel positron emission tomography radioligand to image the peripheral benzodiazepine receptor, a potential biomarker for inflammation. Neuroimage 2008;40(1):43–52.

58. Rusjan P, Wilson AA, Bloomfield PM, et al. Quantification of translocator protein binding in human brain with the novel radioligand, [18F]-FEPPA and positron emission tomography. J Cereb Blood Flow Metab 2011;31(8):1807–16.

59. Guo Q, Colasanti A, Owen DR, et al. Quantification of the specific translocator protein signal of 18F-PBR111 in healthy humans: a genetic polymorphism effect on in vivo binding. J Nucl Med 2013;54(11):1915–23.

60. Ikawa M, Lohith TG, Shrestha S, et al, Biomarkers Consortium Radioligand Project T. 11C-ER176, a radioligand for 18-kDa translocator protein, has adequate sensitivity to robustly image all three affinity genotypes in human brain. J Nucl Med 2017; 58(2):320–5.

61. Jucaite A, Cselenyi Z, Arvidsson A, et al. Kinetic analysis and test-retest variability of the radioligand [11C](R)-PK11195 binding to TSPO in the human brain - a PET study in control subjects. EJNMMI Res 2012;2:15.

62. Collste K, Forsberg A, Varrone A, et al. Test-retest reproducibility of [(11)C]PBR28 binding to TSPO in healthy control subjects. Eur J Nucl Med Mol Imaging 2016;43(1):173–83.

63. Hashimoto K, Inoue O, Suzuki K, et al. Synthesis and evaluation of 11C-PK 11195 for in vivo study of peripheral-type benzodiazepine receptors using positron emission tomography. Ann Nucl Med 1989;3(2):63–71.

64. Setiawan E, Wilson AA, Mizrahi R, et al. Role of translocator protein density, a marker of neuroinflammation, in the brain during major depressive episodes. JAMA Psychiatry 2015;72(3):268–75.

65. Innis RB, Richards E, Pike V, et al. Neuroinflammation in depression: PET imaging of translocator protein (TSPO) and opportunities for COX-1 and COX-2. In: Society of biological psychiatry, vol. 79. Atlanta (GA): Elsevier; 2016. p. 2S–3S.

66. Steiner J, Walter M, Gos T, et al. Severe depression is associated with increased microglial quinolinic acid in subregions of the anterior cingulate gyrus: evidence for an immune-modulated glutamatergic neurotransmission? J Neuroinflammation 2011;8:94.

67. Steiner J, Bielau H, Brisch R, et al. Immunological aspects in the neurobiology of suicide: elevated microglial density in schizophrenia and depression is associated with suicide. J Psychiatr Res 2008; 42(2):151–7.

68. Van Otterloo ES, Miguel-Hidalgo JJ, Stockmeier C, et al. Microglia immunoreactivity is unchanged in the white matter of orbitofrontal cortex in elderly depressed patients. Paper presented at: Society for Neuroscience, 2005; Washington, DC.

69. Kreisl WC, Lyoo CH, McGwier M, et al, Biomarkers Consortium PETRPT. In vivo radioligand binding to translocator protein correlates with severity of Alzheimer's disease. Brain 2013;136(Pt 7):2228–38.

70. Suridjan I, Pollock BG, Verhoeff NP, et al. In-vivo imaging of grey and white matter neuroinflammation in Alzheimer's disease: a positron emission tomography study with a novel radioligand, [F]-FEPPA. Mol Psychiatry 2015;20(12):1579–87.

71. Coughlin JM, Wang Y, Minn I, et al. Imaging of glial cell activation and white matter integrity in brains of active and recently retired national football league players. JAMA Neurol 2017;74(1):67–74.

Moving?

Make sure your subscription moves with you!

To notify us of your new address, find your **Clinics Account Number** (located on your mailing label above your name), and contact customer service at:

Email: journalscustomerservice-usa@elsevier.com

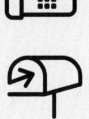

800-654-2452 (subscribers in the U.S. & Canada)
314-447-8871 (subscribers outside of the U.S. & Canada)

Fax number: 314-447-8029

Elsevier Health Sciences Division
Subscription Customer Service
3251 Riverport Lane
Maryland Heights, MO 63043

ELSEVIER

Printed and bound by CPI Group (UK) Ltd, Croydon, CR0 4YY

03/10/2024

01040383-0008